Aids to Pharmacolog

For Churchill Livingstone

Publisher: Timothy Horne
Project Editor: Dilys Jones
Sales Promotion Executive: Marion Pollock

Aids to Pharmacology

Steven Sacks
MB ChB BSc PhD FRCP
Honorary Senior Lecturer, United Medical
and Dental Schools of Guy's and
St Thomas's Hospitals
Consultant Renal Physician,
Guy's Hospital, London

Roy Spector
MD PhD FRCP
Emeritus Professor of Applied Pharmacology,
University of London
Honorary Consultant Physician,
Guy's Hospital, London

THIRD EDITION

CHURCHILL LIVINGSTONE
EDINBURGH LONDON MADRID MELBOURNE NEW YORK AND TOKYO 1993

CHURCHILL LIVINGSTONE
Medical Division of Longman Group UK Limited

Distributed in the United States of America by
Churchill Livingstone Inc., 650 Avenue of the Americas,
New York, N.Y. 10011, and by associated companies,
branches and representatives throughout the world.

First edition 1980
Second edition 1986
Third edition 1993

ISBN 0-443-04695-6

British Library Cataloguing in Publication Data
A catalogue record for this book is available from the British Library.

Library of Congress Cataloging in Publication Data
Sacks, Steven.
    Aids to pharmacology. — 3rd ed. Steven Sacks, Roy Spector.
        p.   cm.
    Rev. ed. of: Aids to pharmacology / Howard Rogers, Roy Spector.
2nd ed. 1986.
    Includes index.
    ISBN 0-443-04695-6
    1. Pharmacology—Handbooks, manuals, etc. 2. Drugs—Handbooks,
manuals, etc.   I. Spector, R. G. (Roy Geoffrey)   II. Rogers, Howard
(Howard John).   Aids to pharmacology.   III. Title.
    [DNLM: 1. Drugs—handbooks.   2. Pharmacology—handbooks.   QV 39
S121a]
    RM301.12S23   1992
    615'.1—dc20
    DNLM/DLC
    for Library of Congress   92-21013

Produced by Longman Singapore Publishers (Pte) Ltd
Printed in Singapore

Preface

Even though pharmacology lies along the borderlands of several sciences (molecular biology and physiology in particular), for medical students and postgraduate doctors it has one outstanding purpose. This is to provide a scientific basis for the sensible use of drugs in human therapeutics.

The purpose of this book is to provide some notes, mainly in list and table form, for revision before preclinical pharmacology examinations in the medical course. The clinical implications of this basic information are given emphasis and it is hoped the book will be of assistance to those preparing for the final MB therapeutics and those postgraduate examinations which require a knowledge of drug action. Students in faculties other than medicine may also find some of the lists and tables a useful summary of the information required in their examinations.

We would like to acknowledge the help of Drs Michael Brada, Rachel Heathcock, Brendan Hicks, Gordon Salden and David Swirsky.

S.S.
R.S.

London, 1993

Contents

1. Introduction

MEDICAL PHARMACOLOGY EXAMINATIONS

The first pharmacology examinations which medical students face are those in the 2nd MB or basic medical sciences part of the MB course. In addition pharmacology crops up in the therapeutics and other parts of the final MB examinations.

In written papers, essay-type questions in pharmacology lend themselves to a systematic approach—even though an absolutely rigid scheme is not possible because there must be few drugs about which everything is known. In writing an essay answer, a homogenous mass of writing can be a depressing sight for the examiner to come across, since it is difficult to see if the main points have been covered. It is far better for the examiner and candidate to have the topic split into separate paragraphs. If a drug or drug group is being discussed, then the following separate paragraphs should be constructed according to the mnemonic **CAME KATE**.

Chemical group (a) whether chemical structure is relevant to actions (e.g. phenothiazines, steroids). (b) any chemical or physical properties which may be relevant (e.g. highly charged, strong base, insoluble, lipid soluble). There is, however, no point in attempting to learn any of this if it has no clinical relevance.

Actions which assign the drug to a particular pharmacological group (e.g. vasodilator, anxiolytic, loop diuretic, anti-arrhythmic of the sodium channel blocking type). This information is always very important. Once the basic pharmacological group of a drug is known, with a little luck the rest of the story can be made up reasonably well.

Mechanisms of action. Not too much is known about this with many drugs, but what is known is often fascinating, e.g. opiates, neuroleptics, anti-inflammatory analgesics, antibacterials, anti-tumour agents.

Even when basic molecular mechanisms are not known, various sites of action may be likely (e.g. limbic system for anxiolytic drugs, loop of Henle for frusemide).

Effects (or pharmacodynamics, or what the drug does to the body).
The candidate (and examiner) should ask what is known about the
spectrum of activities from various points of view.
1. Biochemical (e.g. enzyme inhibition, inducer, uncouples oxidative
   phosphorylation)
2. Physiological (e.g. lowers peripheral resistance, tachycardia)
3. Pharmacological (e.g. local anaesthetic, quinidine-like,
   anticholinergic)
4. Cellular (e.g. cytoxic, arrests cell division, alters membrane
   permeability).
Obviously there is overlap here and it is wise to avoid tedium by not
writing the same information under three or four different headings.

Kinetics: pharmacokinetics (i.e. what the body does to drugs—
including all the factors which govern the concentration of the drug
in the plasma). Many things have to be thought of. Perhaps All
Diets Mean Eating Badly will help.
   Absorption
   Distribution
   Metabolism—are any of the metabolites active?
   Excretion
   Blood—plasma half life, first or zero order pattern of elimination,
   volume of distribution, protein binding, relation of blood levels to
   therapeutics effects and to toxicity.

Applications in clinical medicine.

Toxicity
1. Dose independent (including allergy)
2. Dose dependent
3. Special risks to individual organs and to the fetus
4. Carcinogenicity
5. Addiction.

Effects on the disease process, e.g. arrest of pathological process,
reversibility of lesions, suppression of symptoms,
chemotherapeutic effects.

It is much clearer to write in these headings (and perhaps underline
them) but if the candidate has a modest store of information it is safer
not to label the paragraphs because the omissions will show up too
clearly.
   Naturally some questions will require slight restructuring of this
scheme (e.g. Compare and contrast the intravenous anaesthetics).
Other questions will require great restructure (e.g. How may a
knowledge of pharmacokinetics reduce the risk of drug toxicity?).
Many questions will require the instant construction of a tailor-made
new edifice (e.g. How may the actions of drugs be prolonged?).
   In the MCQ of the London MB the structure of each question is a
stem followed by 5 sub-statements. The candidate has to mark in

(soft black) pencil on the computer answer sheet whether each of the five parts is right or wrong. Because of the general difficulty in setting MCQs, the grammar of the stem and sub-parts often becomes complicated. It is therefore advisable to read the stem twice and then to test each statement by saying (sub-vocally) 'Yes, that's right' or 'no, it isn't' and then mark the answer sheet accordingly. This is particularly helpful when the unfortunate examiner has had to bring in negatives, as for example in the question:

The actions of anticholinesterases such as physostigmine

NO	i.e.	WRONG	A. are not affected by atropine
YES	i.e.	RIGHT	B. are similar to those of acetylcholine
YES	i.e.	RIGHT	C. block the actions of curare
NO	i.e.	WRONG	D. block the actions of suxamethonium
YES	i.e.	RIGHT	E. are not affected by propranolol

The scheme of marking in all the MB examinations with which we are associated is:

a correct part of an answer scores 1 mark
an incorrect part of an answer loses 1 mark
an unanswered part of an answer scores no mark.

Statistically it does not make much difference if you guess or leave blanks if you do not know an answer. In practice it helps to have some insight and only guess when you have some knowledge about the subject and to leave blanks when there is total ignorance.

The viva is a face-to-face confrontation in which the examiner wants to find out what the candidate knows—and, in the great majority of cases, not what he doesn't know. Even with this reassurance it is alarming for the candidate because an answer has to be produced for every question. As a pump-priming measure many examiners ask an easy opening question. ('Do you know any of the actions of histamine?') or a very general one ('What do you know about drug metabolism?'). It is important to start off with simple (but correct) statements rather than anything erudite ('The liver is the most important site of drug metabolism—but it happens in other sites as well', rather than 'cytochrome P_{450} is involved'). Usually the simple easy facts are the most important. If you do not know—according to your own personality—it is worth risking an educated guess. But after one guess, it is then safer to come clean and say you don't know.

During revision, keep an eye on points which some examiners could consider serious errors during a viva and make sure you know these. Several such howlers are not knowing:

classification of muscarinic and nicotinic receptors
classification of α and β adrenergic receptors
route of administration of adrenaline
dangers of isoprenaline

dangers of glucocorticoids
classification of H_1 and H_2 actions of histamine
mode of action of aspirin
food and drug interactions of monoamine oxidase inhibitors
actions of cardiac glycosides
actions of morphine.

Although it is no longer necessary to be as deferential to senior
doctors as in past years, the occasional use of 'Sir' or 'Ma'am' can't
do any harm. Also for males a tie is essential, a haircut and a shave
are desirable and a suit is an advantage. Even though most examiners
are males, women candidates should be adequately covered by
clothing. Bare upper chests and thighs do not usually help. Some of
us have seen it all before.

2. Fundamentals

Pharmacology The science which deals with drugs.
A drug Any substance which changes a physiological function or modifies a disease process.
Therapeutics The science and art of healing disease.
Two types of drugs act on membranes:
Type 1 ('specific') Bind to specific molecules (receptors) in the cell membrane; small alterations in drug structure (even changing the stereoisomerism) can alter drug action (e.g. β agonists or blockers, narcotic analgesics).
Type 2 ('nonspecific') Receptors are not involved but actions depend on the lipid solubility of the drug and its ability to enter cell membranes; alterations in molecular structure which do not alter the drug's physical properties, do not usually greatly change pharmacological effects (e.g. anaesthetics).
Receptor A macromolecular structure which has chemorecognition properties of specific drugs. The binding of such drugs produces a change initiating a chain of events leading to a response by a cell or tissue.
Agonist A drug which can bind to a receptor to produce a response.

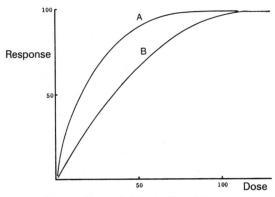

Fig. 2.1 Dose response curve (linear plot) Drugs A and B.

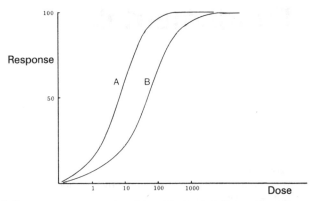

Fig. 2.2 Dose response curve (semi-logarithmic plot). Drugs A and B.

Antagonist A drug which can influence (perhaps by binding to) a receptor and produce no response, although the action of an agonist is prevented.

Dose response curves The axis labelled *dose* is not really drug dose but is its concentration in the liquid surrounding the cell or other structure whose response is being measured. The middle part of the semi-log plot is linear, and therefore gradients and parallelism can be measured.

A and B are both *agonists,* but the potency of B is about one-tenth that of A.

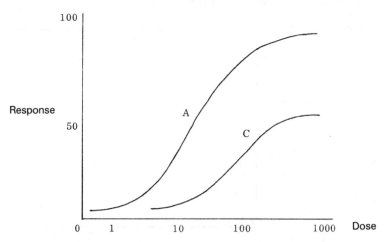

Fig. 2.3 Dose response curve (semi-logarithmic plot). Drugs A and C.

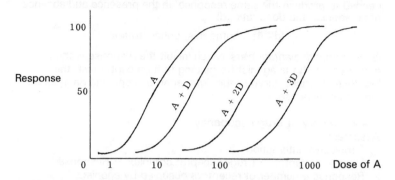

Fig. 2.4 The dose response curve of agonist A in the presence of increasing concentrations of antagonist D.

When the maximal response to drug C is less than that to drug A, C is said to be a *partial agonist*.

An antagonist which acts by binding to the receptor will not affect the maximum response of the agonist, but shifts the dose response curve to the right (see above).

This type of antagonism is called *competitive inhibition*. The degree of antagonism can be expressed as the ratio of the doses of agonist

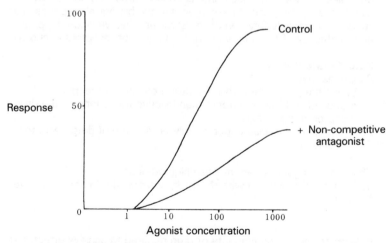

Fig. 2.5 Dose response curve in the presence and absence of a non-competitive antagonist.

needed to produce the same response, in the presence and absence of antagonist: the dose ratio (d).

$$(d - 1) \propto \text{antagonist concentration}$$

Non-competitive antagonists which inhibit the response without competing with the agonist for binding to its receptor shift the log-dose response curve to the right, alter its slope and depress the maximum response.

Clark's theory of drug occupancy
Assumes:
1. Bimolecular interaction
   Drug + Receptor → Drug–Receptor complex → Response
2. Response $\propto$ number of receptors occupied by agonist.

From the law of mass action if p_A is the fraction of receptors occupied, X_A is the agonist concentration and K_A is the equilibrium dissociation constant of the drug—receptor interaction

$$P_A = \frac{X_A}{X_A + K_A}$$

This equation predicts: (a) the shape of the experimentally observed dose response curve and (b) that the potency of a drug (agonist or antagonist) is solely determined by affinity for receptors.

Stephenson's modification of occupation theory
Partial agonists which cannot produce a maximum response regardless of however much drug is applied, are not predicted by Clark's theory. Stephenson assumed that the biological response is a specific but variable function of the stimulus. This variation depends on the efficacy of the drug and on the number of receptors occupied.

Paton's rate theory
Supposes that:
1. When drug combines with receptor a quantum of response is produced and the receptor is then inactive for as long as the drug receptor complex exists.
2. Intensity of response depends only on the rate of drug–receptor combination.

Thus potent agonists can maintain high rates of association/dissociation with receptor; antagonists do not dissociate from receptor.

Tolerance Increasing amounts of drug required to achieve effect, e.g. opiates.

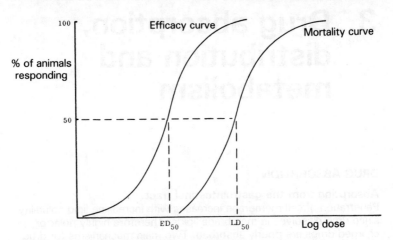

Fig. 2.6 Graph for calculation of therapeutic indices.

Tachyphylaxis Rapidly developing tolerance, e.g. indirectly acting sympathomimetic amines (tyramine, amphetamine), histamine-releasing agents.

$$\textbf{Therapeutic index} = \frac{\text{median lethal dose}}{\text{median effective dose}} = \frac{LD_{50}}{ED_{50}}$$

3. Drug absorption, distribution and metabolism

DRUG ABSORPTION

Absorption from the gastrointestinal tract
Penetration of cell membrane increases with increasing lipid solubility since drug dissolves in membrane lipids. Therefore highly polar or charged drugs are poorly absorbed. Two main mechanisms for drug absorption from gastrointestinal tract
1. *Passive diffusion*—by far the most common
   —obeys Fick's law
   i.e. rate of diffusion $= PA (x_1 - x_2)$
   where P is a permeability coefficient
   A is membrane area
   $(x_1 - x_2)$ is concentration difference across membrane
2. *Active transport*—specific, carrier-mediated, energy dependent mechanism.
   Examples: levodopa, methyldopa, methotrexate, lithium, iodide.

Buccal absorption
Used to decrease extent of hepatic first-pass metabolism for, e.g. nitroglycerine, oxytocin.

Rectal absorption
1. Avoids gastric acid and enzymes
2. May partially avoid hepatic first-pass metabolism
3. Can be used in patients unable to swallow or who are vomiting
4. Sometimes prolongs drug action due to prolonged absorption
5. Absorption relatively rapid.
   Examples: theophylline, indomethacin, diazepam, ergotamine.

Intramuscular injection
1. Best for lipid-soluble drugs or water-soluble drugs with low MW which can pass capillary membrane
2. Absorption improved by exercise of muscle (increases blood flow)
3. Absorption decresed by e.g. haemorrhage, shock, heart failure
4. Muscle sites not identical: absorption from deltoid > absorption from gluteus maximus

5. Can be used to prolong drug action if drug given in viscous, oily vehicle, e.g. fluphenazine decanoate, hydroxyprogesterone injection BP
6. Avoids hepatic first-pass metabolism
7. Can give poor absorption if drug precipitates at injection site, e.g. phenytoin, diazepam.

Intravenous injection
1. Rapid
2. Complete drug availability: avoids hepatic first-pass metabolism
3. Used for drugs unabsorbed orally, e.g. aminoglycosides, or too painful to be given by i.m. injection, e.g. nitrogen mustard.

BIOAVAILABILITY

Definition Extent to which and the rate at which the active substance in a drug product is taken up by the body in a pharmacologically active form.
Bioinequivalence Statistically significant difference in bioavailability of different preparations of the same drug.
Therapeutic inequivalence Clinically significant bioinequivalence. Likely to occur if:
1. Steep dose–response curve
2. Low therapeutic index
3. Dose-dependent (non-linear) pharmacokinetics obeyed (e.g. some preparations of digoxin and phenytoin).

Bioavailability estimated by
1. Comparison with intravenous administration for which bioavailability is 100%
2. Comparison of time to peak plasma concentration between formulations
3. Comparison of peak plasma concentration between formulations
4. Comparison of areas under plasma concentration, time curves.

DRUG DISTRIBUTION

PLASMA PROTEIN BINDING OF DRUGS

Plasma protein binding influences the following:
1. Drug distribution—high MW of plasma protein prevents bound drug from diffusing out of capillaries into tissues
2. Drug effects—free drug fraction is active drug fraction since it can penetrate into region of receptors
3. Drug elimination—free drug is filtered at the glomerulus and excreted into saliva, CSF, milk.

Drug binding is to:
1. Specific carrier protein—relatively unusual, e.g. corticosteroid binding globulin, also binds thyroxine and vitamin B_{12}

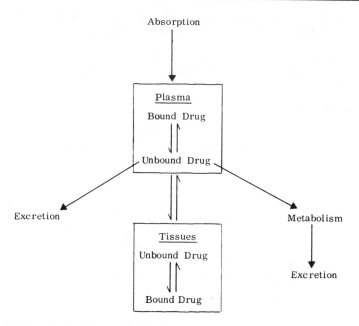

Fig. 3.1 Drug distribution.

2. Albumin—most common binding site for drugs. Albumin concentration in plasma is 4.5 g/100 ml which represents 40% of total body albumin (remainder is extravascular)
3. Acid α_1 glycoprotein—binds basic drugs, e.g. quinidine, imipramine, alprenolol, propranolol, chlorpromazine. This component of plasma increases during inflammatory disease
4. Lipoproteins, e.g. imipramine, quinidine
5. Erythrocytes, e.g. propranolol, quinidine
6. Tissue proteins, e.g. digoxin binds to membrane ATPase.

Drug displacement by competition for binding sites results in the liberation of more drug in the free (active) form.

Examples:

Displaced drug	Displacing drug	Clinical effect
Tolbutamide	Phenylbutazone	Hypoglycaemia
Phenytoin	Salicylate	Phenytoin intoxication
Warfarin	Tolbutamide	Haemorrhage
Endogenous bilirubin	Sulphonamide	Kernicterus

Drug binding decreased by disease states, e.g. liver disease, hypoproteinaemia may result in adverse effects.

DRUG METABOLISM

Drug metabolism chemically modifies drugs and in this way may:
1. Abolish their activity (e.g. *oxidation* of phenytoin, alcohol; *hydrolysis* of suxamethonium, acetylcholine; *conjugation* of isoprenaline, salicylate)
   or
2. Promote or increase activity (e.g. *conversion* of chloral to trichlorethanol)
   or
3. Produce no change in acitivity (e.g. *monodealkylation* of tricyclic antidepressants).

Two phases of metabolism:
Phase I—Metabolic modification (e.g. oxidation, reduction, hydrolysis)
Phase II—Synthesis—i.e. conjugation (e.g. with glucuronic acid, glycine, glutamine, sulphate, acetate)

$$\text{Drug} \xrightarrow[\text{enzymes}]{\substack{\text{Phase I} \\ \text{oxidising etc.}}} \text{metabolites} \xrightarrow[\text{enzymes}]{\substack{\text{Phase II} \\ \text{conjugating}}} \substack{\text{conjugated} \\ \text{metabolites}}$$

PHASE I METABOLISM

1. Smooth endoplasmic reticulum, e.g. barbiturates
2. Cytosol, e.g. ethanol
3. Mitochondria, e.g. oxidation of tyramine.

1. Smooth endoplasmic reticulum
Microsomal oxidation results in:
   a. Aromatic hydroxylation
   b. Aliphatic hydroxylation
   c. N—dealkylation
   d. O—dealkylation
   e. S—oxidation.

Examples

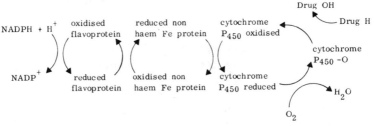

Fig. 3.2

Aromatic hydroxylation:

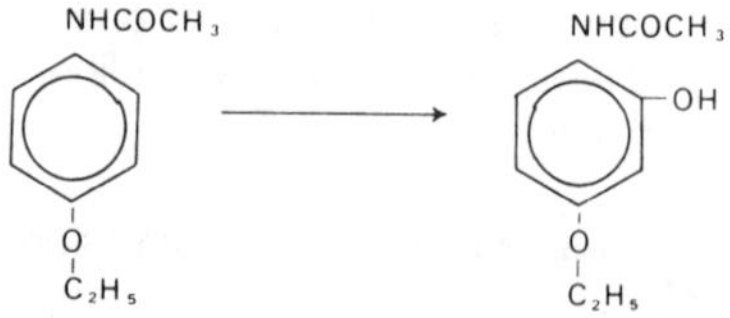

phenacetin   2 hydroxyphenacetin

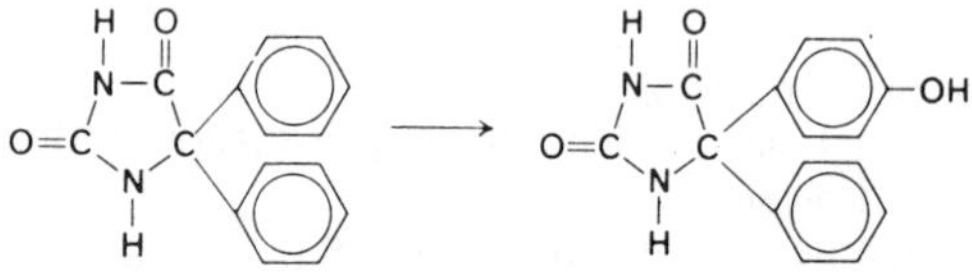

phenytoin   5-(p-hydroxyphenyl)-5-phenylhydantoin

aliphatic hydroxylation:

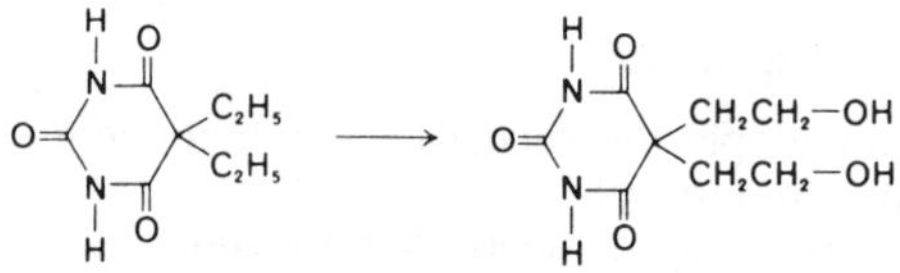

barbitone   inactive hydroxy derivative

N-dealkylation:

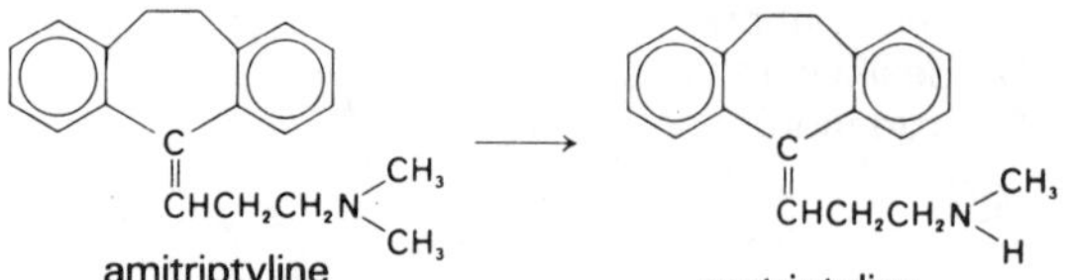

amitriptyline   nortriptyline

O-dealkylation

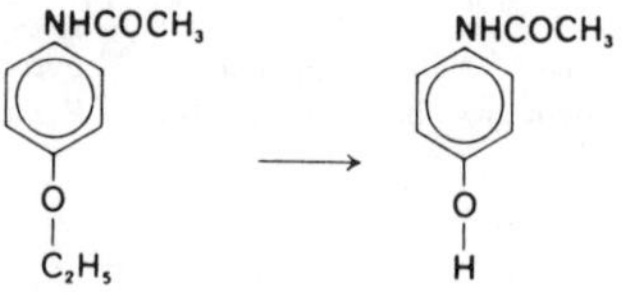

phenacetin   paracetamol

Fig. 3.3

S-oxidation:

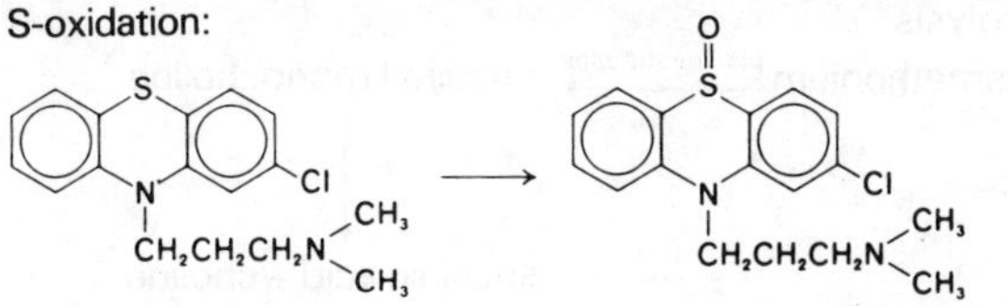

chlorpromazine → chlorpromazine sulphoxide

Fig. 3.3 (contd)

Factors required: NADPH, oxygen, mixed function oxidase and cytochrome P_{450}.

Microsomal reduction
Requires NADPH—cytochrome C reductase
or NADH—cytochrome b_5 reductase

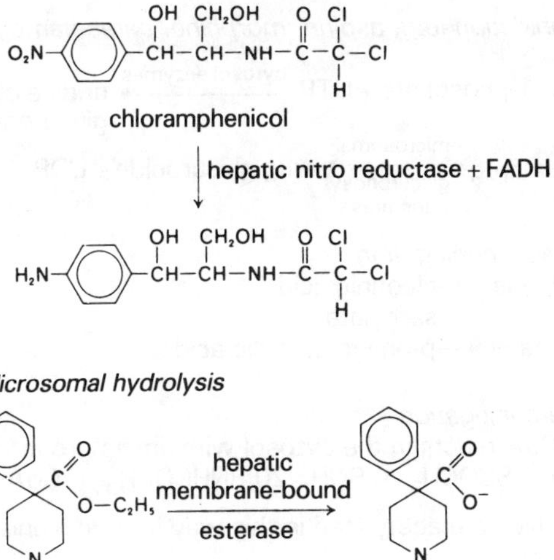

chloramphenicol

hepatic nitro reductase + FADH

Microsomal hydrolysis

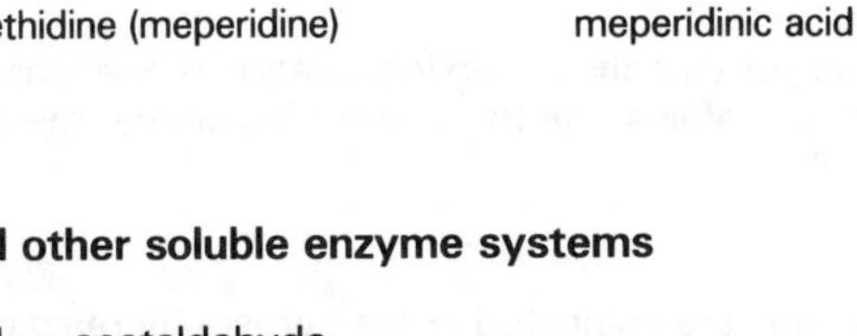

pethidine (meperidine) → meperidinic acid

hepatic membrane-bound esterase

Fig. 3.4

2. Cytosol and other soluble enzyme systems
Oxidation:
ethyl alcohol → acetaldehyde

Hydrolysis:

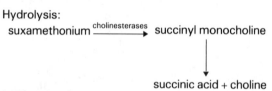

$$suxamethonium \xrightarrow{cholinesterases} succinyl\ monocholine$$

$$\downarrow$$

$$succinic\ acid + choline$$

3. **Mitochondria**
Monoamine oxidase (MAO) and diamine oxidase oxidatively deaminate primary amines to aldehyde or ketones.

Substrates for MAO include catecholamines and tyramine.

Intestinal organisms
These often remove glucuronide groups from conjugated drugs during enterohepatic circulation.
May also be important in metabolism of some drugs, e.g. salicylazosulphapyridine, methotrexate.

PHASE II METABOLISM—CONJUGATIONS

Glucuronidation (e.g. aspirin, morphine, paracetamol)

$$glucose\text{-}1\text{-}phosphate + UTP \xrightarrow{cytosol\ enzymes} \begin{array}{l}uridine\ diphosphate\\glucuronic\ acid\ (UDPGA)\end{array}$$

$$UDPGA + drug \xrightarrow[\substack{glucuronosyl\\transferase}]{microsomal} drug\ glucuronide + UDP$$

Amino acid conjugation
With glycine   —nicotinic acid
                salicylate
With glutamine—p-amino salicylic acid

Acetate conjugation
Acetyl CoA reacts in the cytosol with amine groups of drugs
    $CoA—SCOCH_3 + RNH_2\ 20\ RNHCOCH_3 + CoA—SH$

Drugs which are acetylated in this way include isoniazid and hydralazine.

Methylation
Methyl donor for catecholamine inactivation is S-adenosyl methionine.
Other enzymes catalyse methylation of histamine, mercaptoethanol and thiouracil.

Sulphation
Hydroxyl groups are sulphated in the cytosol by reactions with adenosine-3'-phosphate-5'-phosphosulphate (PAPS).

Ethereal sulphates formed of dihydroandrosterone, oestrone and chloramphenicol

Ribosides and riboside phosphates
Ribonucleosides and ribonucleotides are formed with purine and pyrimidine analogues. Many antimetabolites used in cancer chemotherapy form active metabolites in this way, e.g.:

6-mercaptopurine + 5-phosphoribosyl-1-pyrophosphate (PRPP) →
 6-mercaptopurine nucleoside monophosphate + pyrophosphate.

ENZYME INDUCTION

Enhancement of enzyme activity due to increase in the amount of enzyme protein present in the cell. Induction of enzymes concerned with drug metabolism accelerates the destruction of the drug and reduces their action. The process is usually studied in the liver parenchyma, but it also occurs in other cells, e.g. fibroblasts, lymphocytes.

Three groups of inducing agents
1. Substances which stimulate metabolism in many pathways, e.g. barbiturates.
2. Polycyclic hydrocarbons (e.g. 3-methyl cholanthrene; 3-4 benzo (a) pyrine).
   These produce limited metabolic stimulation.
3. Steroids: mainly microsomal enzyme stimulation.

Effects of enzyme inducing substances on metabolism of endogenous and exogenous chemicals

Enzyme inducing agent	Substances whose metabolism is enhanced
Barbiturates	Barbiturates, warfarin, phenytoin, contraceptive pill, digitoxin, chlorpromazine, phenylbutazone, cortisol, testosterone, bilirubin, vitamin D_3, folic acid, tricyclic antidepressants
Phenytoin and carbamazepine	Digitoxin, thyroxine, dieldrin, DDT, steroids, anticonvulsants, contraceptive pill, vitamin D_3, folic acid
Ethanol	Ethanol, warfarin, phenytoin, barbiturates, tolbutamide
DDT, gamma benzene hexachloride	Cortisol, phenytoin, phenazone
Aldrin, dieldrin, endrin	Widespread acceleration of drug metabolism
Phenazone	Bilirubin, warfarin, cortisol
Griseofulvin	Warfarin
Rifampicin	Contraceptive pill, warfarin, rifampicin

Smoking accelerates the metabolism of:
   nicotine
   dextropropoxyphene and other analgesics
   tricyclic antidepressants
   theophylline.

Inhibition of drug metabolism

Drug	Substance whose metabolism is inhibited
Isoniazid	Phenytoin
Chloramphenicol	Phenytoin, tolbutamide
Sodium valproate	Anticonvulsants
Ethanol (single large dose)	Chloral, tolbutamide, phenytoin, warfarin
Coumarins	Tolbutamide
Disulphiram	
Sulphonylureas	
Metronidazole	Acetaldehyde (from ethanol)
Procarbazine	

Environmental inducers
 1. 3-methyl-cholanthrene and other polycyclic aromatic
    hydrocarbons
 2. Urea herbicides
 3. Volatile oils
 4. Dyes
 5. Nicotine and other alkaloids
 6. Preservatives
 7. Safrole
 8. Xanthines (including caffeine)
 9. Flavones
10. Organic peroxides.

Environmental inhibitors of microsomal enzymes
1. Organophosphorus insecticides
2. Pesticide synergists (methylene dioxyphenly derivatives)
3. Carbon tetrachloride
4. Ozone
5. Carbon monoxide.

First pass metabolism
Drug metabolism after oral administration but before drug enters the
systemic circulation so that a significant fraction of the drug is
inactivated before it becomes available to the whole body. Occurs to
a variable degree between drugs and between individuals. May be
important cause of interindividual variation.

1. First-pass metabolism in intestinal mucosa: methyldopa, levodopa, chlorpromazine, tyramine, clorazepate, stilboestrol, testosterone, progesterone
2. First-pass metabolism in the liver: propranolol, labetalol, oxprenolol, lignocaine, glyceryl trinitrate, pethidine, pentazocine, imipramine, nortriptyline, amitriptyline, prazepam
3. First-pass metabolism in the bronchial mucosa (of inhaled drugs): isoprenaline, nicotine.

First-pass metabolism may result in drugs being unavailable if given by some routes (e.g. glyceryl trinitrate orally); or they may produce

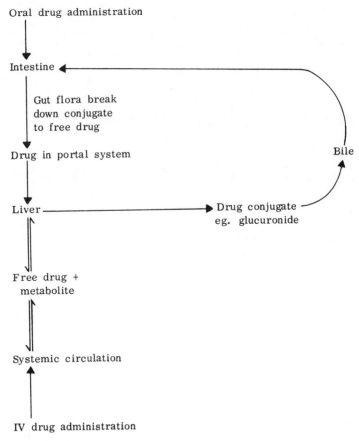

Fig. 3.5 Enterohepatic circulation.

different metabolites when administered by some routes (e.g. 4-hydroxypropranolol is formed after oral but not i.v. administration).

ENTEROHEPATIC CIRCULATION (FIG. 3.5)

Examples: throxine, phenolphthalein, carbenoxelone, contraceptive pill, refampicin.

4. Pharmacokinetics

Definition
Study of the time course of drug absorption, distribution, metabolism and excretion (ADME) and of the mathematical relationships required in modelling this data.

Compartmental models
These consider the body as a series of well-stirred compartments into each of which the administered drug simultaneously distributes. The simplest model is that the body is a single compartment.

First order elimination kinetics
The rate of a process is proportional to the amount of drug present (just as the rate of emptying of a bath depends upon the amount of water in it). Sometimes called *linear kinetics* because it is described by linear differential equations. If X is the amount of drug in the body

$$-\frac{dX}{dt} \propto X$$ i.e. rate of elimination is proportional to the amount of drug present

then

$$-\frac{dX}{dt} = kX$$ (minus because the amount of drug is decreasing)

where k is the first order rate constant (i.e. a proportionality constant).

For a one compartment model of the body, if an amount of drug X_0 is administered and eliminated by a first order process and the rate constant for elimination is k (units, time^{-1})

$$\frac{dX}{dt} = -kX$$

Integrating gives

$$X_t = X_0 e^{-kt}$$

where X_t is amount of drug in the body at time t (Analogous to other familiar exponential processes, e.g. discharge of an electrical condenser).

Amount of drug, $X \propto$ concentration of drug in body C

$$X = V_d C$$

V_d is a proportionality constant with the units of volume called the apparent volume of distribution. It has no physiological or anatomical connotation and for some drugs may be very large, e.g. for imipramine and nortriptyline it is about 50 l/kg body weight. V_d depends upon

1. Drug factors, e.g. lipophilicity, protein binding
2. Patient factors, e.g. body weight, plasma proteins
3. The pharmacokinetic model assumed.

Thus $C_t = C_0 e^{-kt}$ which plotted on linear coordinates gives:

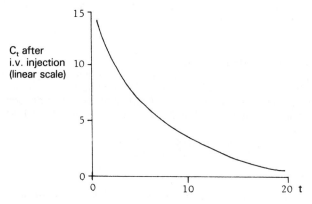

Fig. 4.1

This can be linearised by plotting log C_t against time:

$$\log C_t = \log C_0 - \frac{kt}{2.303}$$

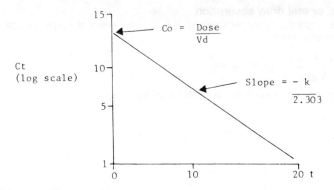

Fig. 4.2

$$V_d = \frac{X_0}{C_0} = \frac{dose}{C_0}$$

$$= \frac{X_0}{k\,(AUC)}$$

where AUC = area under plasma concentration, time curve.

Half life
Time for drug concentration in the plasma to decline by one-half.

$$t_{\frac{1}{2}} = \frac{0.693}{k}$$

Total body clearance
A more accurate measure of the efficiency with which drug is eliminated by the body than $t_{\frac{1}{2}}$. Defined as the portion of the V_d cleared of drug in unit time. It has units of flow (ml per min).

$$Cl = kV_d$$

$$= \frac{0.693V_d}{t_{\frac{1}{2}}}$$

$$= \frac{X_0}{AUC}$$

Total body clearance = sum of the clearance by each eliminating organ (e.g. liver, kidneys).

I.m. or oral drug absorption

In a single compartment model: if k_a = first order absorption rate constant, then

$$C_t = \frac{k_a F X_0}{V_d(k_a - k)} \, (e^{-kt} - e^{-k_a t})$$

where F is the systemic availability of the drug

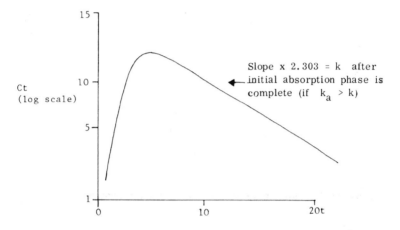

Slope x 2.303 = k after initial absorption phase is complete (if k_a > k)

Fig. 4.3

NB V_d cannot be determined by back extrapolation to find C_0 in this case.

Two compartment models of the type

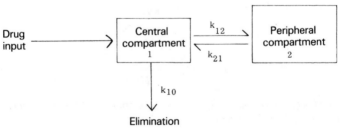

Fig. 4.4

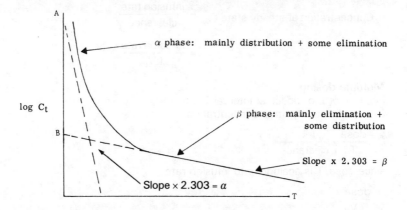

Fig. 4.5 Plasma levels in two compartment model.

For i.v. injection: $C_t = Ae^{-\alpha t} + Be^{-\beta t}$

$$t_{\frac{1}{2}}\beta = \frac{0.693}{\beta}$$

V_d may take different values depending upon the part of the blood level curve under consideration.

Bioavailability fraction
Comparison made by reference to either:
1. Intravenous dose (100% available) *or*
2. Standard oral preparation

$$\text{Apparent availability F} = \frac{\left(\int_0^\infty C\,dt\right) \text{oral}}{\left(\int_0^\infty C\,dt\right) \text{i.v.}}$$

$$= \frac{(AUC)\ \text{oral}}{(AUC)\ \text{i.v.}}$$

$F = F_{\text{(completeness of absorption)}} \times F_{\text{(first-pass metabolism)}}$

If absorption is complete, F estimates the magnitudes of first-pass metabolism.

Constant i.v. infusion
The amount of drug in the body increases up to a plateau level when the amount of drug infused equals the amount of drug lost from the body in unit time.

$$\text{Concentration at steady state } C_{ss} = \frac{\text{infusion rate}}{\text{clearance}}$$

$$= \frac{\text{infusion rate}}{kV_d}$$

Multiple dosing
I.v., i.m. or p.o. doses at interval T
$\bar{C}$ = mean steady state concentration

$$\bar{C} = \frac{\text{dose}}{T} \times \frac{1}{\text{clearance}}$$

since dose/T is analogous to infusion rate

$$= \frac{\text{dose}}{TkV_d}$$

as $k = 0.693/t_{1/2}$ and $1/0.693 = 1.44$

$$\bar{C} = \frac{1.44 \times \text{dose} \times t_{1/2}}{V_d T}$$

If $F < 1$

$$\bar{C} = \frac{1.44F \times \text{dose } t_{1/2}}{V_d T}$$

Assuming $F = 1$ and constant V_d during multiple dosing, a drug will accumulate in the body if it is given at intervals less than 1.4 times its half-life. The ratio of accumulation is defined as

$$R = \frac{1.4t_{1/2}}{T}$$

$$= \frac{\bar{C}}{\text{dose}}$$

i.e. R defines by what multiple $\bar{C}$ exceeds the amount given in a single dose, For a given dose it is possible to calculate the valueo of T necessary to achieve a desired $\bar{C}$ from $T = AUC/\bar{C}$.

Time to reach steady state
When amount administered during dosage interval = amount eliminated during dosage interval, this is *solely* dependent upon $t_{1/2}$. On a repeated dosage regimen after $5 \times t_{1/2}$, 97% of the steady state level has been attained. Conversely after $5 \times t_{1/2}$, 97% $(1 - 0.5^5)$ of the drug originally in the body has been eliminated after administration has ceased.

Loading dose can be used to achieve steady state more rapidly.

$$\text{Loading dose, L} = \frac{\text{Maintenance dose}}{1 - e^{-kT}}$$

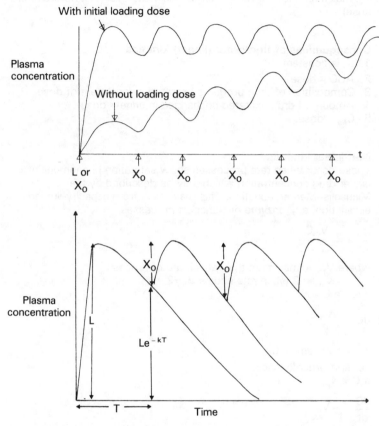

Fig. 4.6 Plasma drug concentrations resulting from administration of loading dose L followed by repeated maintenance doses X_0 at dosing interval T, so $L = X_0 + Le^{-kT}$.

Fluctuations in blood levels when plateau is reached:
  Maximum level – Minimum level = Dose/Vd

$$\frac{C_{max}}{C_{min}} = 2^{(T/t\frac{1}{2})}$$

e.g. if doses are given every 2 half-lives

$$\frac{C_{max}}{C_{min}} = 2^2 = 4$$

i.e. maximum blood level is 4 times minimum level (just before next dose).

Consequences of first order (linear) kinetics
1. $t_{1/2}$ is constant
2. AUC $\propto$ dose
3. Composition of drug products excreted independent of dose
4. Amount of drug excreted unchanged in urine $\propto$ dose
5. $C_{ss} \propto$ dose.

Non-linear kinetics
These occur when rate processes show saturation phenomena at higher drug concentration which may be described by the Michaelis–Menten equation. This may result from capacity-limited elimination, e.g. enzyme or transport processes.

$$\frac{dC}{dt} = - \frac{V_m C}{K_m + C}$$

where V_m = maximum theoretical rate of process
$\quad\quad K_m$ = C when rate equals $V_m/2$
If $K_m \gg C$

$$\frac{dC}{dt} = - \frac{V_m C}{K_m}$$

$$= \text{constant} \times C$$

i.e. first-order kinetics.
If $C \gg K_m$

$$\frac{dC}{dt} = - V_m$$

$$= \text{constant}$$

i.e. zero order kinetics: the rate is independent of drug concentration.
    On log-linear coordinates a curved line describes the decline in plasma concentration with time.

Consequences of non-linear kinetics
1. Decline of C with t is not exponential
2. $t_{1/2}$ increase with dose
3. AUC is not proportion to dose

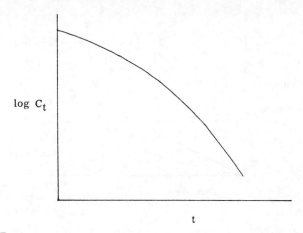

Fig. 4.7

For zero order kinetics in linear coordinates:

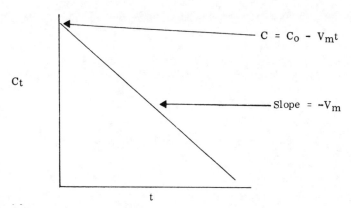

$C = C_0 - V_m t$

$Slope = -V_m$

Fig. 4.8

4. Composition of excreted products affected by dose
5. Amount of unchanged drug excreted in urine is not proportional to dose
6. Possibility of drug–drug interactions due to competition for some capacity limited process
7. On multiple dosing disproportionate increases in steady state levels occur with small increases in maintenance dose.

$$C_{ss} = \frac{K_m \times Dose}{V_m - Dose}$$

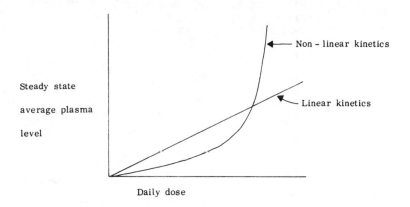

Fig. 4.9

Examples of drugs obeying non-linear kinetics:
Ethanol, salicylate, phenytoin and overdoses of tricyclic
antidepressants and benzodiazepines.

5. Pharmacogenetics

Genetic influences can result from a single mutant gene (producing discontinuous variation) or polygenic influences (producing continuous variation).

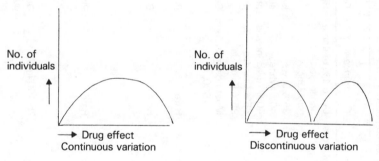

Fig. 5.1

Genetic variation can affect drug metabolism (Table 5.2) or drug responsiveness (Table 5.3).

Table 5.1 Incidence of acetylator status

Genotype and acetylator status		Europeans	Eskimos and Japanese	Mediterranean Jews
E^aE^a E^ae^a	rapid acetylators	40–45%	95%	20–35%
e^ae^a	slow aceylators	55–60%	5%	65–80%

Clinically important with:
1. Isoniazid
2. Procainamide
3. Hydralazine

Table 5.2 Variations in drug metabolism due to genetic polymorphism

Pharmacogenetic variation	Mechanism	Inheritance	Occurrence	Drugs involved	Effect
Acatalasia	Lack of r.b.c. catalase	Autosomal recessive	Up to 1% of some Japanese populations	Hydrogen peroxide	Approx. 50% suffer recurrent sepsis of mouth and pharynx
Rapid acetylator status	Increased hepatic acetylase	Autosomal dominant	35% Jews 40% whites 40% Asian Indians 85% Chinese 95% Eskimos	Isoniazid, hydralazine, some sulphonamides, phenelzine, procainamide.	↑ dose requirement; ↓ response; generally ↑ toxicity
Suxamethonium sensitivity	Several types of abnormal plasma pseudocholinesterase	Autosomal recessive	Most common form 1:2500	Suxamethonium	Prolonged muscle relaxation following suxamethonium
Failure to metabolise phenytoin	Deficiency of phenytoin 5-phenyl hydroxylase	Autosomal or X-linked dominant	Rare	Phenytoin	Phenytoin toxicity in usual doses
Coumarin sensitivity	Deficiency of a mixed function hepatic microsomal enzyme which oxidises bishydroxycoumarin	Unknown	Rare	Bishydroxycoumarin	Excess anticoagulation may lead to haemorrhage
Phenacetin-induced methaemoglobinaemia	Deficiency of mixed function hepatic de-ethylating microsomal enzyme	Autosomal recessive	Rare	Phenacetin	Methaemoglobinaemia
Defective alicyclic hydroxylation	Unknown	Unknown	?5:100 in UK	Debrisoquine, guanoxan, phenacetin, encainide, perhexilene, some β-blockers	Individual variation in dose needed for therapeutic response

Table 5.3 Variation in drug response due to genetic polymorphism

Pharmacogenetic variation	Mechanism	Inheritance	Occurrence	Drugs involved
G6PD deficiency: favism, drug-induced haemolytic anaemia	80 distinct forms of G6PD. Chronic deficit of reduced SH groups exacerbated by administration of oxidising drugs	X-linked incomplete codominant	10 000 000 affected in the world. Probably protects against malaria	Many—including 8-aminoquinolines, antimicrobials and minor analgesics (see text)
Steroid-induced raised intraocular pressure	Unknown	Autosomal recessive (heterozygotes show some response)	5% white population	Glucocorticoids (see text)
Warfarin resistance	Reduced affinity of vitamin K epoxide reductase of warfarin	Autosomal dominant	Rare	Warfarin
Haemoglobin Zurich: sulphonamide induced haemolysis	Arginine substituted for histidine at 63rd position of β chain of haemoglobin	Autosomal dominant	Rare	Sulphonamides
Haemoglobin H: drug-induced haemolysis	Haemoglobin composed of four β chains	Autosomal recessive	1:300 births in Bangkok	Same drugs as for G6PD deficiency
Methaemoglobinaemia: drug-induced haemolysis	Methaemoglobin reductase deficiency	Autosomal recessive (heterozygotes show some response)	1:100 are heterozygotes	Same drugs as for G6PD deficiency

(contd)

Table 5.3 (contd)

Pharmacogenetic variation	Mechanism	Inheritance	Occurrence	Drugs involved
Malignant hyperthermia with muscular rigidity	Unknown	Autosomal dominant	1:20 000 of population	Some anaesthetics, especially halothane. Also suxamethonium
Inability of taste phenylthiourea or phenylthiocarbamide	Unknown	Autosomal recessive	1:3 of whites	Drugs containing the N–C=S group such as thiouracils
Porphyria: exacerbation induced by drugs	Increased activity of δ-amino levulinic acid synthetase exacerbated by drugs due to inherited enzyme deficiencies in the pathway of haem synthesis	Autosomal dominant	Acute intermittent type 15:1 000 000 in Sweden; Porphyria cutanea tarda 1:100 in Afrikaaners	Barbiturates, chloral, chloroquine, ethanol, sulphonamides, phenytoin, griseofulvin (see text)

4. Dapsone
5. Sulphamethazine and some other sulphonamides
6. Sulphasalazine
7. Phenelzine.

Suxamethonium sensitivity

Genotype	Phenotype	Prevalence	Response to suxamethonium
$E_1^u E_1^u$	Usual type of esterase	94%	Normal
$E_1^a E_1^a$	Atypical esterase dibucaine resistant	1:2500	Grossly prolonged
$E_1^f E_1^f$	Fluoride resistant	Rare	Prolonged
$E_1^s E_1^s$	Silent. No enzyme activity	1:100 000	Grossly prolonged
$E_1^u E_1^a$	Heterozygote pattern	1:25	Normal (or almost normal)
$E_1^u E_1^f$	Heterozygote pattern		Normal (or almost normal)
$E_1^a E_1^f$	Heterozygote pattern		Prolonged
$E_1^u E_1^s$	Heterozygote pattern	1:200	Almost normal
$E_1^a E_1^s$	Heterozygote pattern	1:80 000	Grossly prolonged

A high activity cholinesterase designated E_{cyn}, produces suxamethonium resistance.

Table 5.4 Steroid-induced raised intraocular pressure

Increase in intraocular pressure on exposure to 0.1% dexamethasone eye drops (mm Hg)	0–5	5–15	15+
Percentage of population	66	29	5
Proposed genotype	$p^L p^L$	$p^L p^H$	$p^H p^H$
Chance of ultimate development of open angle glaucoma in later life (compared with $p^L p^L$ individuals)	1	18	101

Subjects with G6PD deficiency may develop haemolysis when exposed to:

1. *Analgesics*—aspirin, phenacetin, acetanilide, antipyrene, aminopyrine
2. *Antimalarials*—primaquine, pamaquine, pentaquine, quinacrine, quinine
3. *Antibacterials*—sulphonamides, sulphones, nitrofurantoin, chloramphenicol, PAS
4. *Miscellaneous*—quinidine, probenecid, BAL, vitamin K, naphthalene.

Mechanism

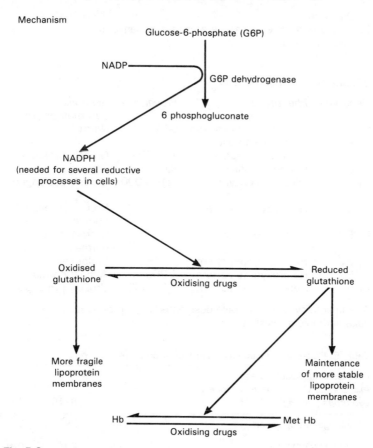

Fig. 5.2

The porphyrias

Neurological (pain, paralysis, coma) —in acute intermittent and variegate porphyrias

Psychiatric (e.g. mania) —in acute intermittent and variegate porphyrias

Cardiovascular —in acute intermittent porphyria

Gastrointestinal (e.g. abdominal pain) —in acute intermittent porphyria

Photosensitivity —in variegate porphyria and hereditary coproporphyria

Increased urinary porphobilinogen —in acute intermittent porphyria

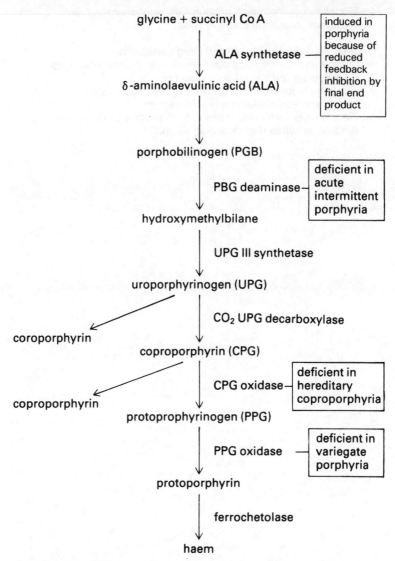

Fig. 5.3 Haem synthesis showing various enzyme defects in the porphyrias.

Acute exacerbations precipitated by:
1. *Hypnosedatives*—barbiturates, dichloralphenazone, benzodiazepines
2. *Anticonvulsants*—phenytoin, succinimides
3. *Oral hypoglycaemics*—sulphonylureas

4. *Miscellaneous*—ethanol, griseofulvin, sulphonamides, sex hormones, oral contraceptive pills.

Genetic disorders with altered drug sensitivity
1. *Down's syndrome:* excessive sensitivity to anticholinergics
2. *Gout aggravated by:* ethanol, diuretics
3. *Gilbert's disease:* helped by barbiturates; aggravated by oestrogens and cholecystographic agents
4. *Transketolase deficiency:* prone to Wernicke and Korsakoff syndromes when dependent on alcohol.

6. Transmitters in the peripheral and central nervous systems

NEUROTRANSMITTERS

Neurotransmitters are substances secreted by a nerve which impart information to specific targets (receptors) in cells.

Classical neurotransmitters
Rapidly open ion channels causing depolarisation or hyperpolarisation.

Non-classical neurotransmitters
Reduce ion conductance causing depolarisation or hyperpolarisation. These act on leak channels which are open in some resting neurones.

Neuromodulators
Slowly enhance or suppress depolarisation or hyperpolarisation caused by neurotransmitters. Examples are some peptides and aminoacids which have only small postjunctional effects on their own but, like classical transmitters, are released from neuronal storage vesicles.

Neurohormones
These are secreted into the blood from some neurones when depolarised. Certain hypothalamic neurones also release their hormones (oxytocin, ADH) as neurotransmitters into synapses.

Neuromediators
These are substances which are formed in response to transmitter stimulation. They participate in the production of transmitter actions and include such second messengers as cyclic AMP and cyclic GMP.

Neurones were thought to secrete only one transmitter, but it now seems that a neurone may secrete two or more transmitters—perhaps some of them modulate the actions of classical transmitters liberated at the same time.

Responses to classical transmitters are of three types
1. Increased permeability to Na^+ or Ca^{++} causing depolarisation (excitatory postsynaptic potential; EPSP)

2. Increased permeability to anions (esp. Cl′) causing
   hyperpolarisation (inhibitory postsynaptic potential; IPSP)
3. Increased permeability to K⁺, allowing outflow of K⁺ and thus
   hyperpolarisation (IPSP).

When EPSP exceed the threshold then an action potential results.
Inhibitory transmitters produce IPSP which reduces EPSP and reduces
the chance of triggering an action potential.

TRANSMITTERS IN THE PERIPHERAL NERVOUS SYSTEM

Site	Transmitter (receptor)	Antagonist
Sympathetic and parasympathetic autonomic ganglia	Acetylcholine (nicotinic) (M_1 muscarinic)	Hexamethonium Pirenzepine
Sympathetic neuroeffector junctions	Noradrenaline (α adrenoceptor) (β adrenoceptor)	Phenoxybenzamine Propranolol
Parasympathetic neuroeffector junctions	Acetylcholine (muscarinic)	Atropine
Motor end plate (voluntary nervous system)	Acetylcholine (nicotinic)	Curare

Parasympathetic autonomic system
Cranio-sacral outflow

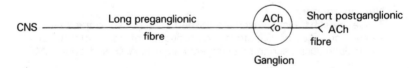

Fig. 6.1

Sympathetic autonomic system
$T_1 - L_2$ outflow

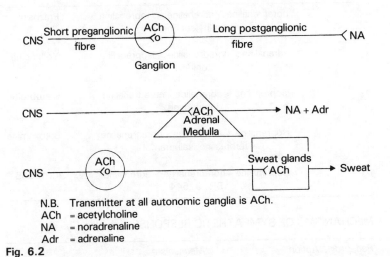

N.B.   Transmitter at all autonomic ganglia is ACh.
ACh   = acetylcholine
NA   = noradrenaline
Adr   = adrenaline

Fig. 6.2

SYMPATHOMIMETIC AMINE ACTIONS
(classified according to adrenoceptor type)

α_1	α_2	β_1	β_2	β_3
Contraction of vascular and genitourinary smooth muscle	Decreased neuronal release of noradrenaline	Increased heart rate, contractility and conduction velocity	Relaxation of vascular bronchial and alimentary smooth muscle	Stimulation of lipolysis in fat
Relaxation of intestinal smooth muscle	Platelet aggregation	Renin release	Tremor	
	Reduced insulin release		Glycogenolysis and gluconeogenesis in liver	
	(possible contraction of vascular smooth muscle)			

AGONISTS AND ANTAGONISTS OF ADRENOCEPTORS

Receptor	Agonists	Antagonists
α_1	noradrenaline > adrenaline > isoprenaline phenylephrine	Prazosin
α_2	adrenaline > noradrenaline > isoprenaline clonidine	Yohimbine
β_1	isoprenaline > adrenaline = noradrenaline dobutamine	Metoprolol
β_2	isoprenaline > adrenaline > noradrenaline terbutaline, salbutamol	Butoxamine
β_3	isoprenaline = noradrenaline > adrenaline BRL 37544	ICI 118551

MECHANISMS OF SYMPATHETIC RESPONSE (see also Ch. 7)

Receptor	Action	Mechanism
α_1	Contraction of smooth muscle	Stimulation of phospholipase C causes hydrolysis of membrane phospholipid to diacylglycerol (DAG) and inositol triphosphate (IP3) Increase in cytosol Ca^{++}
α_1	Intestinal relaxation	Opening of K^+ channels causes hyperpolarisation
α_2	Decreased release of NA from nerves	Closure of Ca^{++} channels
α_2	Contraction of vascular smooth muscle	Ca^{++} influx
α_2	Reduced insulin release	Inhibition of adenyl cyclase
β_1	All actions	Activation of adenyl cyclase and opening of Ca^{++} channels
β_2	All actions	Activation of adenyl cyclase
β_3	Lipolysis in adipose tissue	Activation of adenyl cyclase

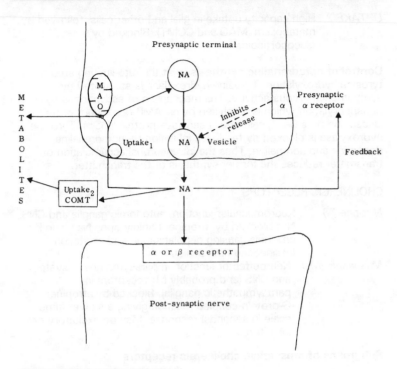

ADRENERGIC NERVE TERMINAL
NA = Noradrenaline
COMT = Catechol—O—methyl transferase
MAO = Monoamine oxidase

Fig. 6.3

NB Phenoxybenzamine blocks pre- and postsynaptic α receptors
Prazosin blocks only postsynaptic α receptors
Clonidine stimulates presynaptic α receptors
Mianserin blocks presynaptic α receptors

Termination of actions of noradrenaline and adrenaline
UPTAKE 1 High affinity, high specificity, low capacity active
reuptake in noradrenergic fibres. Blocked by tricyclic
antidepressants and cocaine

UPTAKE 2   High capacity uptake in glial and other cells, followed by metabolism (MAO and COMT). Blocked by glucocorticoids

Control of noradrenaline synthesis is at the rate-limiting step of tyrosine hydroxylation. Tyrosine hydroxylase is stimulated by sympathetic nervous activity. The mechanism of activation is by phosphorylation which is catalysed by an AMP-dependent protein kinase and by a Ca^{++} calmodulin-sensitive protein kinase. Tyrosine hydroxylase is blocked by feedback inhibition by noradrenaline, dopamine and adrenaline. Thus the intraneuronal accumulation of transmitter reduces the further synthesis of the transmitter.

CHOLINERGIC RECEPTORS

Nicotine (N)   Neuromuscular junction, autonomic ganglia and CNS. Not blocked by atropine. Rapidly open Na^+ and K^+ channels causing depolarisation and excitation (millisecond time scale).

Muscarinic (M_1)   Neuroeffector junction in parasympathetic system and CNS (and probably M_1 receptors in parasympathetic ganglia). Blocked by atropine. G-protein-coupled reaction giving a slower (time scale in seconds) response. May be excitatory or inhibitory.

Subgroups of muscarinic cholinergic receptors

Receptor type	Antagonist	Site	Mechanism
M_1	Pirenzepine Atropine	Some glands (esp. gastric) or the ganglia innervating them (causing secretion) CNS	Receptors stimulate G proteins, which activate phospholipase. Thus DAG and IP_3 formed which increase Ca^{++} in cytosol and cause depolarisation
M_2	Atropine	Heart (slows SA firing and slows conduction)	Opens K^+ channels, inhibits adenyl cyclase
M_3	Atropine Hexahydrosiladifenol	Smooth muscle (contraction) Some glands (secretion)	Stimulation of phospholipase C thus raising DAG and IP_3. Increased cytosol Ca^{++}

Competitive inhibitors of muscarinic cholinergic receptors

Drug	Special features and uses
Atropine (dl-hyoscyamine)	Central stimulant in overdose. Used for: premedication, in the treatment of sinus bradycardia, organophosphorus and mushroom poisoning, side effects of anticholinesterases, symptomatic treatment of diarrhoea, local mydriatic (recovery 7–10 days)
Hyoscine (scopolamine)	Sedative. Used for premedication and sea sickness. Local mydriatic (recovery 3–7 days)
Homatropine	Weaker and shorter action than atropine. Only used locally as a mydriatic (recovery 1–3 days)
Cyclopentolate	Local mydriatic (recovery 1 day)
Tropicamide	Local mydriatic (recovery 6 hours)
Propantheline	Powerfully antimuscarinic. Weakly ganglion blocking. Used to reduce smooth muscle spasm and to reduce gastric secretion in peptic ulcer disease
Poldine	Similar to propantheline

Acetylcholine (ACh) production by neurones

$$\text{Choline} + \text{acetyl CoA} \xrightarrow[\substack{\text{choline acetyltransferase} \\ \text{(CAT)}}]{} \text{ACh}$$

Final synthetic step in vesicles in axon terminals.

CAT synthesised in perikaryon with other neuronal proteins, then transported along axon. Axon terminals contain mitochondria in which acetyl CoA is synthesised.

One action potential causes release of 100 or more quanta (vesicles) of ACh
One vesicle contains 1000–50 000 molecules of ACh
One motor neurone terminal has 300 000 or more vesicles
One ACh molecule causes a potential change of 3×10^{-7} volts
Miniature end plate potentials (mepps) are due to constant release of quanta of ACh in sub threshold amounts
Cardiac and smooth muscle have spontaneous activity due to rhythmical fluctuations of membrane potentials which trigger action potentials. This is pacemaker activity. In intestinal smooth muscle ACh increases spike frequency (by Ca^{++} mobilisation) but slows the heart (by raising potassium permeability).

Termination of ACh action is by membrane-bound
acetylcholinesterase. Anticholinesterases block this and thus increase
cholinergic activity. Reversible anticholinesterases (e.g. neostigmine
and pyridostigmine) used to raise ACh level at motor end plate in
treatment of myasthenia gravis and to reverse curare-like drugs.
   Irreversible anticholinesterases (e.g. parathion and malathion) are
used as insecticides.

Cholinergic effects via automatic nervous system

1. Cardiovascular   Slows heart rate and AV conduction
                    Cholinergic sympathetic vasodilation in striated
                    muscle
                    Congestion and erection of sex organs
2. Lungs   Bronchiolar constriction and bronchial secretion
3. Glands   Sweating (sympathetic cholinergic)
                    Increased secretion by stomach, intestine, lacrimal
                    and salivary glands
4. Eye   Miosis and accommodation for near vision
5. Smooth muscle   Intestinal peristalsis, relaxation sphincters
                    Contraction of bladder.

CENTRAL NERVOUS SYSTEM TRANSMITTERS

Acetycholine
Both muscarinic (M) and nicotinic (N) receptors in the CNS:

Receptor	Agonist	Antagonist	Action
M_1	Muscarine	Pirenzepine	Excitatory
		Atropine	
M_2	Bethanechol	Atropine	Inhibitory
N	Nicotine	Dihydro β-erythroidine	Excitatory

Renshaw cells are N cholinergic neurones in the anterior horn of the
cord which modulate motoneurone activity. Both N and M neurones
are found in the following long divergent projections and local circuits:
medial septal nucleus → dentate gyrus ⎫ memory and
subiculum of hippocampus → interpendicular nucleus ⎬ cognitive
⎭ function

cortical interneurones → cortical pyramidal neurones ⎫ control and
thalamus, putamen, caudate → caudate neurones ⎬ modulation of
⎭ movement

Alzheimer's dementia is associated with degeneration of cholinergic
neurones in the hippocampal region and connections. Attempts at
treatment include cholinergic agonists (e.g. pilocarpine) and
anticholinesterases (e.g. physostigmine).

CATECHOLAMINES (DOPAMINE, NORADRENALINE, ADRENALINE)
Dopamine (DA; D)

Receptor	Agonist	Antagonist	Action	Mechanism
D_1	Dopamine 15 × more active on D_1 than on D_2	SCH 23390	Inhibitory	Activates adenyl cyclase
D_2	Apomorphine	Sulpiride Butyrophenones	Inhibitory	Not linked with adenyl cyclase

Dopaminergic neurones
Ultrashort in retina and olfactory bulb
Intermediate from ventral hypothalamus to pituitary (inhibits prolactin
    release); chemoreceptor trigger zone to vomiting centre
Long projections: substantia nigra → striatum (control of movement)
                   ventral tegmentum → amygdala and other parts of
                   the limbic system (expression and memory of
                   emotional experiences).
    Antipsychotic drugs act by blocking D_2 receptors in the limbic
system. Blocking of D receptors in the extrapyramidal system causes
movement disorders. Blockade of D receptors in the chemoreceptor
trigger zone is antiemetic.

Noradrenaline (NA)
Both α and β receptors are in the CNS. Central actions of NA depend
on pre-existing activity of target neurones (i.e. NA effects are
modulatory or state-dependent). At α receptors NA inhibits neuronal
firing; at β receptors it either inhibits or excites, but usually increases
rate of firing via a cAMP mechanism which inhibits K^+ conductance.
    NA present in hypothalamus and parts of the limbic system. Most
NA neurones in locus coeruleus of pons and also in lateral tegmentum
of reticular formation. These give rise to axonal radiations to cortical,
subcortical and brain stem regions. These multiple branching
radiations appear to be concerned with emotional arousal.
    Many antidepressant drugs enhance NA actions by blocking
reuptake 1 of NA or by modulating receptor responsiveness to NA.
However other amines such as 5HT and DA are also enhanced by
these drugs.

Adrenaline
Adrenaline containing neurones are relatively few in the CNS, being
mainly restricted to the medullary reticular formation. These neurones
radiate to pontine nuclei and paraventricular nuclei of the dorsal
midline thalamus.
    Adrenaline is here possibly involved in integration of autonomic
responses.

5-hydroxytryptamine (5HT; serotonin)
Six central 5HT receptors have been described:

Receptor	Actions
$5HT_1$ (subtypes A, B, C, D)	Inhibitory. Activates adenyl cyclase
$5HT_2$	Excitatory. Activates phospholipase C
$5HT_3$	Excitatory

Inhibitory actions are due to hyperpolarisation caused by increased K^+ conductance; excitation is due to depolarisation caused by reduced K^+ conductance.

Many 5HT neurones travel rostrally and caudally from râphé nuclei. Importance ascending 5HT pathways are:

rostral râphé nuclei → limbic system (inhibition)
dorsal râphé nuclei → cerebral cortex (excitation)

The râphé systems inhibit sensory input and thus perhaps govern limbic (emotional) responses to external stimuli.

LSD may be hallucinogenic due to inhibition of râphé activity and therefore allows different stimuli to overactivate the limbic system.

5HT itself inhibits the firing of râphé 5HT neurones and thus could increase limbic responses. Antidepressants of the lofepramine type block uptake 1 of 5HT and could thus act by râphé inhibition.

Central blockade of 5HT actions increases appetite and lofepramine type drugs reduce appetite and can cause nausea.

The peripheral $5HT_1$ agonist sumatriptan acts in migraine by constricting the cerebral arteries. However when applied intracerebrally it inhibits 5HT release.

Histamine (H)
Three types of histamine receptors have been described in the CNS. These probably have an excitatory action. The receptors are on neurones, but H_1 receptors have also been found in glia and cerebral blood vessels.

Receptor	Antagonist	Mechanism
H_1	Chlorpheniramine	Mobilisation of Ca^{++}
H_2	Cimetidine	Activates adenyl cyclase
H_3	Thioperamide	Unknown

Most H neurones are in the ventral posterior hypothalamus, from which arise long caudal and rostral tracts. Histamine appears to mediate arousal and wakefulness. H_1 antihistamines such as chlorpheniramine produce sedation; only those with little CNS penetration (e.g. terfenadine and astemizole) do not usually cause sleepiness.

AMINO ACIDS

Excitatory and inhibiting amino acids are widespread in the brain. Excitatory amino acids include the dicarboxylic acids glutamate and aspartate. The monocarboxylic ω-amino acids (GABA, glycine, β-alanine, taurine) are inhibitory.

Glutamate and aspartate

These are powerful excitatory transmitters found in almost every region of the CNS and are involved in fast synaptic transmission. They may also regulate the permeability of ionic channels which are primarily voltage-dependent. There are three types of receptor for these stimulatory amino acids:

Receptor	Agonists (in addition to glutamate and aspartate)	Antagonists
KAI	Kainic acid (from seaweed) is 50 × more potent than glutamate, although it damages nerves	Lactonised kainate
QUIS	Quisqualate	Cyanonitroquinoxaline (CNXQ)
NMDA	N-methyl D-aspartame	Carboxypiperazine (CPP) Aminophonovalerate (APV) Argiotoxin 636 (a spider venom)

NMDA receptors are mainly present on spinal cord excitatory neurones.

The voltage-dependent ionic channels which are regulated by NMDA receptors are blocked by ketamine (a dissociative anaesthetic) and the hallucinogen phencyclidine (PCP; angel dust).

Gamma aminobutyric acid (GABA)

GABA mediates inhibitory actions of interneurones in the brain (GABA$_A$ receptors) and is a presynaptic inhibitor (via GABA$_B$ receptors) in the cord. GABA$_A$ produces hyperpolarisation by opening the chloride channel (an example of a ligand-gated channel).

GABAergic inhibitory neuronal projections in the brain include:

cerebellar Purkinje cells → Deiter's nucleus
caudate nucleus → substantia nigra

GABA is also found in the cerebral cortex, cuneate nucleus, hippocampus and lateral septal nucleus.

Directly or indirectly bicuculline, picrotoxin, pentylenetetrazol and penicillin antagonise GABA receptors and thus cause CNS stimulation and fits. Some antiepileptic drugs—vigabatrin and valproate—act by inhibiting the metabolic breakdown of GABA.

The anti-anxiety drugs, the benzodiazepines bind to GABA receptor-chloride channel complex and facilitate the opening of the channel in the presence of GABA.

Baclofen reduces muscle spasm by stimulating $GABA_B$ receptors which inhibit the release of excitatory transmitters in the cord.

Glycine

Glycine is a central inhibitor in the reticular formation and in the anterior grey horn of the cord. It causes hyperpolarisation by opening chloride channels.

Strychnine causes CNS stimulation and muscular spasms by reducing the hyperpolarisation caused by glycine and β-alanine.

PEPTIDES

Substance P

Substance P is found in afferent sensory fibres, posterior root ganglia and in the posterior grey region of the cord and is involved in transmission of nociceptive stimuli from the periphery.

Other peptides

Encephalins are in the interneurones of the cord in the substantia gelatinosa and antagonises (i.e. has a gating action on) the transmission of nociceptive impulses. They antagonise the release and effects of substance P.

Many peptides originally discovered in the alimentary tract or endocrine system have subsequently been found in the CNS as members of families of structurally related substances. For example the endorphin family now includes proopiomelanocortin, proenkephalin and prodynorphin. The endorphin family appears to be part of the corticotrophin family.

The glucagon family includes glucagon, vasoactive intestinal peptide (VIP) and secretin.

Apart from substance P, several other neuroactive peptides are present in sensory neurones. These are VIP, somatostatin and cholecystokinin.

Non-adrenergic non-cholinergic (NANC)

This term was originally used to describe nerve endings in the peripheral nervous system. The transmitters include purines. However some NANC transmitters such as nitric oxide are in the brain and peripheral nervous system. It mediates gastric relaxation after receiving food.

γ-interferon, interleukin 1-β and endotoxin induce nitric oxide synthase. Nitric oxide activates cGMP and potassium conductance.

7. Receptor structure and mechanisms

The binding of an agonist (ligand) to a receptor causes the production of a regulatory signal either by a direct intracellular effect or by promoting the synthesis or release of another intracellular substance called the second messenger. Although many agonists have been recognised the structural types of receptor appear to be limited. These are exemplified by the cholinergic nicotinic receptor (ligand gated ionic channel); the cholinergic muscarinic receptor (coupled with G protein); growth hormone receptor (protein kinases); glucocorticoid receptor (intracellular soluble protein).

Nicotinic (N) receptor

The N receptors are ligand-gated ionic channels. This means that on attachment of the nicotinic agonist, ionic channels open rapidly causing increased permeability to Na^+ and K^+. Depolarisation and excitation result. There is a direct connection between the ligand site and the ionic channel as the same protein mass is involved. The N receptor is made up of pentameric proteins with at least 2 subunits. Each subunit has several membrane-spanning regions (probably 4). The individual subunits surround an ionic channel. One of the subunits (α) is present in 2 copies and forms the ligand binding site of the receptor. Muscle N receptors have 4 subunits in a pentameric complex (α_2, β, γ). N receptors in the CNS are also pentamers but are built of only α and β.

Other ligand-gated ionic channels

These have a similar structure to the N receptor with several subunits each with many membrane-spanning sequences around a central ion channel. $GABA_A$, glutamate, aspartate and glycine are receptors of this type.

Voltage-gated channels

These are similar to the above and have α and β subunits. The α unit is a helix with projecting charges. An alteration in surrounding potential causes a conformational change which alters the ion channel.

Muscarine (M) receptor

M receptors are glycoproteins with a MW of about 80 000. Analysis of the hydrophobicity of the amino acid sequences predicts they cross the membrane 7 times.

The M receptor is G protein-linked and only affects K^+ and Ca^{++} channels indirectly because the receptor and ion channels are separate proteins; information is exchanged by guanine nucleoside binding regulatory protein (G protein).

Other G protein coupled receptors

These are also folded up as 7 membrane-spanning α helices. When a ligand binds to the receptor, it induces conformational changes on the cytoplasmic face to the G protein. The ligands acting this way are the α_1, α_2, and β-adrenergic agonists, eicosanoids and some peptide hormones.

G protein system

The consequence of combination of a ligand with a G protein-associated receptor is increased binding of GTP to G protein. This activates the G protein which then can do several things:

increased or decreased activity of adenyl cyclase
increased activity of phospholipases C and A_2
opens Ca^{++}, K^+ or Na^+ channels
activates some transport proteins.

Phosphorylated tyrosine systems

Receptors for peptide hormones which regulate growth, differentiation and development are protein kinases which phosphorylate tyrosyl residues. Kinases and guanyl cyclases are globular proteins which occupy the full thickness of the plasma membrane and have ligand (external) and catalytic (cytoplasmic) regions. A single α helix connects the two.

The mediators which act via this system are growth hormones, insulin, oncogene products, including epidermal growth factor, platelet-derived growth factor and some lymphokines.

Intracellular receptors

Steroids, thyroid hormones, vitamin D and retinoids bind to intracellular receptors. These are soluble DNA-binding proteins that regulate the transcription of specific genes (via mRNA production). The binding of the ligand to the carboxy end of the protein allows the central zone to bind to a regulatory region of DNA and activate the adjacent gene. This sequence of steps occupies a prolonged time. For example, in treating severe asthma or anaphyllaxis with glucocorticoids, an initial response may not be discernible for 2–3 hours and the peak benefit is about 24 hours after steroid administration.

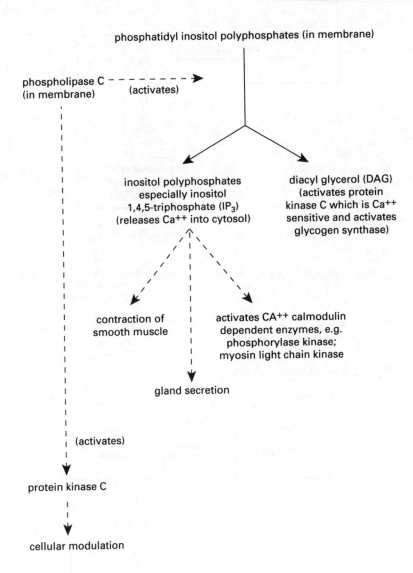

Fig. 7.1 Role of phospholipase C.

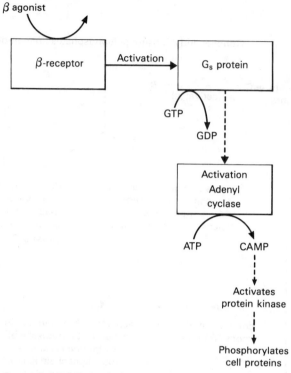

Fig. 7.2 β receptor and G protein.

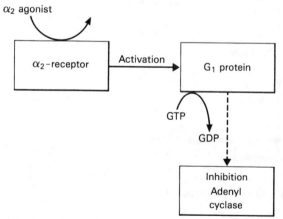

Fig. 7.3 α_2 receptor and G protein.

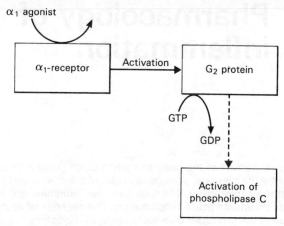

Fig. 7.4 α_1 receptor and G protein.

Presynaptic receptors

There are receptors on the prejunctional neuronal membrane which influence the release of transmitter from the same neurone. The clearest understood of these is the prejunctional noradrenaline receptor (an α_2 receptor) which when stimulated, inhibits the release of noradrenaline.

Prejunctional cholinergic receptors are also found on noradrenergic nerve fibres which, on stimulation, reduce the release of noradrenaline.

Prejunctional M receptors act at cholinergic muscarinic junctions and inhibit depolarisation-mediated release of acetylcholine. Because of such a mechanism, anticholinesterases reduce acetylcholine release, and muscarinic anatagonists enhance it.

Regulation of receptors

The sensitivity of receptors to agonists can vary in either direction. In asthma, the bronchodilator response to β agonists may diminish on repeated administration. Conversely on withdrawal of β blockers the heart may beat rapidly and irregularly due to increased sensitivity of the heart β receptors.

The development of abnormal muscular movements (tardive dyskinesia) in patients who have received long term neuroleptic treatment is in part at least due to supersensitivity of dopamine receptors in the extrapyramidal system caused by prolonged dopamine receptor blockade.

8. Pharmacology of inflammation

The early responses of the body to injury include general effects mediated by the nervous, vascular and reticular systems and local effects at the site of injury. The local vascular, exudative and cellular responses constitute acute inflammation. The changes of acute inflammation are produced by a wide range of mediators:

membrane lipid derivatives (eicosanoids and platelet activating factor)
histamine and other amines
lymphokines
kinins
neutrophil derivatives
complement system.

EICOSANOIDS (eekosi is Greek for 20)

Eicosanoids are derived from 20 C essential fatty acids with 3, 4 or 5 double bonds—arising mainly from membrane arachidonic acid.
   Eicosanoids are not stored, but released from all cell types. The group includes prostaglandins (PGD, PGE, PGF), prostacyclins (e.g. PGI_2) thromboxanes (e.g. TXA_2) and leukotrienes (LTB_4, LTC_4, LTD_4). They act via receptor-associated G proteins.

Synthesis
Arachidonic acid is liberated from membrane phospholipids by the action of phospholipase A_2, which is activated by Ca^{++} and calmodulin. Phospholipase is inhibited by drugs which reduce the availability of Ca^{++} and by glucocorticoids which induce the synthesis of a protein lipocortin which blocks phospholipase activity.
   Aspirin and other non-steroidal anti-inflammatory drugs block the synthesis prostaglandins and thromboxanes by inhibition of cyclooxygenase.
   Physical stimuli activate the entire system by causing an inflow of Ca^{++} which initially accelerates arachidonic acid formation.

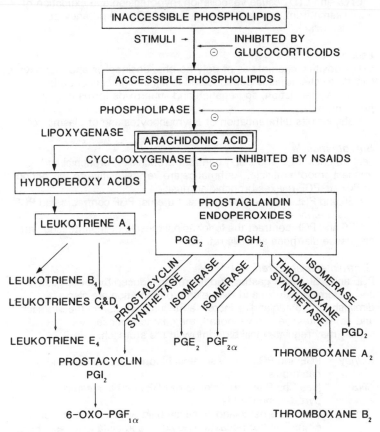

Fig. 8.1 Genesis of prostaglandins and other eicosanoids.

Actions

Vascular system
PGE is a potent dilator of arterioles, precapillaries, postcapillary venules, vascular sphincters. The blood pressure is lowered and the blood flow in viscera is increased.

   PGD_2 vasodilates at low concentration and vasoconstricts at high concentrations.

   PGD_2 and PGF_2 constrict pulmonary arteries and veins

   TXA_2 is a potent vasoconstrictor and aggregator of platelets

   PGI is a vasodilator and lowers blood pressure (with reflex tachycardia), and endothelial PGI_2 inhibits platelet aggregation.

LTC_4 and LTD_4 cause vasodilation, hypotension and exudation of plasma from postcapillary venules (1000 × the potency of histamine).

Leucocytes
LTB_4: positive chemotaxis of polymorphs, eosinophils and monocytes (similar to chemotactic peptides and PAF). In high concentrations causes degranulation, aggregation and superoxide formation by polymorphs.
PGE_2 inhibits differentiation of *B* lymphocytes and of plasma cells.

Smooth muscle
Leukotrienes, PGF and PGD_2 contract bronchiolar, bronchial and tracheal smooth muscle. Asthmatics are very sensitive to this action of $PGF_2\alpha$. PGE relaxes bronchiolar muscle.
PGF and PGE contract the pregnant uterus; PGF contracts and PGE relaxes the non-pregnant uterus.
PGF and PGE contract the longitudinal muscle of the intestine and can cause diarrhoea and bile reflux.

Gastrointestinal secretion
PGE and PGI_2 inhibit gastric acid secretion induced by food, gastrin and histamine. Pepsin and the volume of secretion are also diminished. Prostaglandins increase mucus secretion in the stomach and small intestine and vasodilate the gastric mucosa.
PGI_2 may regulate local blood flow in the stomach.

Kidney	PGE and PGI_2 increase renal blood flow, diuresis and natriuresis
CNS	(see Chs 6 and 7) Release of PGE_2 perhaps causes pyrogen-induced fever
Pain	Injected prostaglandins cause pain which is not immediate or intense but outlasts bradykinin and histamine pain. PGE, PGI_2 and LTB_4 produce hyperalgesia by sensitising afferent nerve endings to chemical and physical stimuli.

PLATELET ACTIVATING FACTOR (PAF)

PAF is a lipid product of membrane phospholipid. It is not stored but released from leucocytes, platelets, endothelial cells, renal mesangial and medullary cells. It is synthesised in response to antigen–antibody combination, chemotactic peptides, thrombin and exposed collagen. PAF itself stimulates PAF synthesis. Synthesis requires phospholipase, acetyltransferase and Ca^{++} and is inhibited by steroids. PAF receptors are linked to G proteins.
PAF contracts smooth muscle including bronchioles and uterus. It is a powerful vasodilator and stimulates platelet and polymorph aggregation, causing the liberation of LTB_4 from these. It also

stimulates the aggregation of monocytes and eosinophils and is chemotactic for eosinophils, monocytes and polymorphs. Gastric ulceration is produced. Although it is a general vasodilator, blood flow to the kidney is reduced. Vascular permeability is increased and like prostaglandins and leukotrienes, it causes hyperalgesia.

HISTAMINE

Histamine is an endogenous substance which is synthesised, stored and released mainly by mast cells, but also by basophils and neurones. It is distributed throughout the body but is in highest concentrations in skin, lungs and alimentary mucosa.

Mast cells and basophils release histamine in the presence of the polyamine 48/80 and morphine. Antigen and IgE cause the release of histamine with PGD_2 and LTC_4. Release is inhibited by sodium cromoglycate, β agonists and glucocorticoids.

Antigen–antibody stimulation of mast cells activates a membrane G protein which enables phospholipase C to form lysophosphatidyl choline and lysophosphatidic acid. This causes fusion of storage granule membrane with plasma membrane, allowing histamine release.

Histamine is one of the mediators of the immediate hypersensitivity reaction of acute inflammation, is involved in gastric acid secretion and in CNS transmission.

There are at least 2 histamine receptors, H_1 and H_2. Their actions can be summarised:

H_1 only	H_1 and H_2	H_2 only
Increased permeability of post-capillary venules; constriction of coronary and basilar arteries; arteriolar dilatation in face; bronchoconstriction	Dilatation of arterioles and venules in limbs; pain and itching	Gastric acid and pepsin secretion; dilatation of arterioles in gastric mucosa; heart-increased rate, force and automaticity; inhibition of IgE-dependent degranulation of mast cells.

H_1 antagonists

These are used for allergic rhinitis, urticaria and motion sickness. Their properties include:
1. CNS depression. But some (e.g. astemizole and terfenadine) are not sedating because they do not penetrate into the CNS
2. Anticholinergic—may contribute to antiemetic (e.g. cyclizine and dimenhydrinate) and anti-Parkinsonian (e.g. orphenadrine) actions. Causes dry mouth
3. Anti 5HT (e.g. cyproheptadine) contributes to antiallergic effects. Increases appetite.

5HT (SEROTONIN)

5HT is another amine which mediates inflammation. It is stored in platelets—human mast cells lack 5HT. It is released from some carcinoid tumours causing attacks of flushing, bronchoconstriction, diarrhoea and endocardial thickening.

5HT initially relaxes then contracts vascular smooth muscle and may be involved in migraine. Some antimigraine drugs (such as pizotifen and methysergide) are 5HT antagonists. Sumatriptan is a selective $5HT_1$ agonist and terminates migraine attacks by constricting cerebral vessels.

LYMPHOKINES

Lymphokines are soluble products released by lymphocytes. T lymphocyte factors include γ interferon (γ IFN) and interleukin 2 (IL-2). IL-2 is a T cell growth factor secreted by helper cells. IL-3 is a multipotential colony stimulating factor. One form of this stimulates polymorphs and monocytes.

Other lymphokines are B cell growth factor, B cell diffusion factor, macrophage activating factor, γ interferon, suppression and helper factors, transfer factor and lymphotoxin. With γ interferon, lymphotoxin can kill cells including cancer cells.

KININS

These are physiologically active peptides which contract smooth muscle. Bradykinin is a non apeptide which is 10 times more active a vasodilator than histamine. It also produces pain and increases vascular permeability, but is not chemotactic to white cells.

The action of kinins is terminated by kininases—one of which is angiotensin I converting enzyme.

Kallikrein forms bradykinin from high MW kininogen. It also activates the Hageman factor (factor XII) to factor XIIa and is chemotactic to leucocytes. C1 esterase inhibitor is a kallikrein inhibitor. When deficient it is associated with a proneness to angioedema. α_1 antitrypsin, another kallikrein inhibitor, may also be lacking in some patients and is associated with hepatic fibrosis in infancy and emphysema in adult life.

NEUTROPHIL DERIVATIVES

Cationic proteins	Increase vascular permeability; neutrophil immobilisation; histamine release; monocyte chemotaxis
Acid proteases	Act on kininogen to form kinin

Neutral proteases   Degrade collagen, basement membrane and fibrin,
cleave C3 and C5 to form active products
Catalyse kininogen → kinin
Increase vascular permeability.

COMPLEMENT SYSTEM

Activation of the complement system forms the anaphylotoxins C_{3a} and C_{5a} which can release histamine from mast cells. C_{5a} is a potent chemotactic factor, as is activated complex C_{567}.

Plasmin has a complex action:
conversion of kininogen to kinin
activation of prekallikrein to kallikrein
activation of C_3 complement to form C_{3a}.

9. Immunosuppressive agents

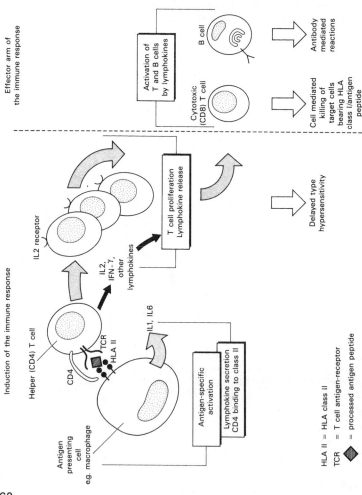

Fig. 9.1 Induction of the immune response. Activation of lymphocytes is dependent on antigen-specific recognition by helper T cells and on various co-factors including lymphokines and accessory molecules, e.g. CD4.

Induction of the immune response

Effector arm of the immune response

Antigen presenting cell e.g. macrophage

Helper (CD4) T cell

IL2 receptor

CD4

TCR

HLA II

IL1, IL6

IL2, IFN-γ, other lymphokines

Antigen-specific activation

Lymphokine secretion CD4 binding to class II

T cell proliferation Lymphokine release

Delayed type hypersensitivity

Activation of T and B cells by lymphokines

B cell

Cytotoxic (CD8) T cell

Antibody mediated reactions

Cell mediated killing of target cells bearing HLA class I/antigen peptide

HLA II = HLA class II
TCR = T cell antigen-receptor
◆ = processed antigen peptide

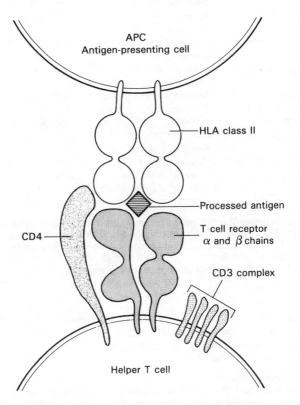

Fig. 9.2 Molecular interactions between an antigen-presenting cell (APC) and a helper T cell, showing the target molecules for anti-CD3 and anti-CD4 monoclonal antibodies. The CD3 complex is involved in signal transduction from the T cell receptor to the interior of the cell. Binding of the CD4 molecule to the framework structure of the HLA class II molecule improves the affinity of the interaction between the APC and the T cell.

Table 9.1 Immunosuppressive agents

Group	Examples	Main action
1. Glucocorticoids	Prednisolone Methylprednisolone	(1); (3), in large doses; anti-inflammatory
2. Antimetabolites	Azathioprine Methotrexate	(2)
3. Alkylating agents	Cyclophosphamide Chlorambucil	(2)
4. Fungal peptides	Cyclosporin A FK506*	(1)
5. Polyclonal immunoglobulin	Antilymphocytic globulin Antithymocytic globulin	(3); (4)
6. Monoclonal antibodies	Anti-CD3 Anti-CD4* Anti-IL2 receptor*	(3); (4)
7. Physical methods	Plasmapheresis Immunoadsorption Total lymphoid irradiation	(5) (5) (1); (2); (3)

* Under clinical evaluation
(1) Inhibit synthesis of lymphokines required for activation of T and B cells;
(2) Inhibit DNA synthesis and therefore prevent replication of lymphocytes;
(3) Block T cell functions dependent on target antigen due to masking, internalisation or shedding of target antigen; (4) Deplete T cells by lysis or enhanced removal by the reticuloendothelial system; (5) Removes circulating antibody.

Uses
1. Autoimmune disease, e.g. SLE, vasculitis, rheumatoid arthritis, glomerulonephritis, psoriasis
2. Allergy, e.g. asthma, contact dermatitis
3. Organ transplantation.

Combination therapy
Agents with different sites of action may be used together to achieve more potent immunosuppression with sparing of side effects of individual drugs. However complications due to the level of immunosuppression are increased.

Complications due to immunosuppression
1. Infections—with common organisms and atypical organisms. The latter include:
   —bacteria (e.g. TB)
   —viruses (e.g. herpes, cytomegalovirus),
   —fungi (e.g. candida, aspergillus, mucor)
   —protozoa (e.g. *Pneumocystis carinii*)
2. Malignancy:
   —Skin cancer
   —lymphoma
   —cervical premalignancy

3. Inhibition of cell division (some agents only):
    —hair loss
    —cytopenia
    —infertility

PREDNISOLONE

Action
Blocks activation of IL1 and IL6 genes in macrophages. Secondary reduction of IL2 synthesis. The immune response is thus dampened at an early stage of activation. Lymphocytotoxic in large doses. General anti-inflammatory effect.

Administration
Oral. Absorption with enteric-coated preparations very variable. High dose intravenous methyl prednisolone may be given.

Uses
Alone (e.g. asthma) or with other immunosuppressive drugs (e.g. systemic vasculitis; transplantation).

Toxicity
Complications are frequent with prolonged use. Common side effects are: diabetes mellitus; obesity; mood changes; osteoporosis; aseptic necrosis of bone; muscle wasting; impaired healing; hypertension and oedema. Growth retardation in children and suppression of the pituitary-adrenal axis; less marked with alternate day prednisolone regimens.

AZATHIOPRINE

Action
Metabolized in liver to 6-mercaptopurine and then to its active metabolite 6-thioinosinic acid. It inhibits DNA and RNA synthesis by preventing synthesis of adenylic acid and guanylic acid from inosinic acid and so blocks T cell proliferation.

Uses
Blocks late in the pathway of T cell activation and so it is usually necessary to give with other immunosuppressive agents such as prednisolone. Used in SLE as a 'steroid sparing' agent, and in transplantation with prednisolone and cyclosporin.

Toxicity
Myelosuppression. Concomitant use of allopurinol is highly dangerous since catabolism of azathioprine by xanthine oxidase is inhibited. This can cause profound neutropenia and over-immunosuppression. Hepatic dysfunction.

CYCLOPHOSPHAMIDE

Action
Covalently binds to DNA, inhibiting DNA replication and cell proliferation. May have some specificity for B lymphocytes.

Uses
With prednisolone in antibody mediated vasculitis. Also for humoral rejection of organ transplants.

Toxicity
Severe myelosuppression, infertility, bladder irritation and cancer (see under Anticancer drugs). To minimise infertility, treatment is preferably limited to two courses of 12 weeks each.

CYCLOSPORIN A (CyA)

Product of the fungus *Trichoderma polysporum*. Cyclic peptide of 11 amino acids.

Action
Completely blocks T cell proliferation by inhibition of activation of IL2 and other lymphokine genes probably due to the inactivation of an isomerase now called cyclophilin. (FK506, a metabolite of *Streptomyces tsukubansis* with promising immunosuppressive effects, has a similar mechanism of action).

Kinetics
The drug is lipid soluble and variably absorbed by mouth so that a period of intravenous loading may therefore be necessary. After an oral dose, blood levels peak in 2–4 h and trough in 12–16 h. Metabolised by liver cytochrome P450.

Uses
Major use in transplantation of kidney, liver, heart, heart–lung and pancreas. Combined with prednisolone, or prednisolone and azathioprine ('triple therapy'). May also be of value in glomerulonephritis, psoriasis.

Toxicity
Marked nephrotoxicity. Hirsutism, shakes, gum hypertrophy. Metabolic-hyperkalaemia, hypomagnesaemia, hyperuricaemia, hyperlipidaemia. Blood CyA levels are increased by drugs which impair hepatic metabolism of CyA. (e.g. erythromycin, fluconazole, diltiazem) and decreased by drugs which enhance hepatic metabolism of CyA (e.g. phenytoin, sodium valproate, rifampicin, isoniazid).

Blood levels
Measured at trough. No precise correlation with clinical function or toxicity. Changes in level or extremes of variation more useful.

ALG AND ATG

Antilymphocytic globulin is raised in horses against cultured lymphoblasts (mainly B cells). Antithymocytic globulin is raised in rabbits against human thymocytes.

Action
Antibody binds to lymphocytes. Reduces lymphocyte count by complement mediated lysis and enhanced cell clearance, and blocks T cell proliferation.

Use
Prevention and treatment of rejection of transplanted organs.

Toxicity
Neutropenia and thrombocytopenia due to contaminating antibody specificities. Allergic-type reactions.

Other limitations
Batch variability arising from the mix of antibodies.

MONOCLONAL ANTI-CD3 (OKT3)

Mouse monoclonal antibody raised against human T lymphocytes.

Action
Binds to the delta chain of the tetramolecular CD3 complex associated with the α/β receptor of T cells. Causes early depletion of lymphocytes due to enhanced clearance and possibly complement mediated lysis. Prolonged therapy is associated with loss of expression of CD3/TCR complex on the cell surface (modulation). This may be due to internalization or shedding of target antigen.

Use
Treatment or (less commonly) prevention of transplant rejection. Severe vasculitis resistant to drug therapy.

Toxicity
'Flu-like symptoms with first or second dose associated with cytokine release; can be dampened by glucocorticoid given concomitantly. Pulmonary oedema due to capillary leak. Neutropenia.

10. Drugs affecting the central nervous system I. Psychotropic drugs and neurology

PSYCHOTROPIC DRUGS

Anti-anxiety agents (anxiolytics, sedatives, minor tranquillisers)
Hypnotics
Antipsychotic drugs (neuroleptics, major tranquillisers)
Antidepressants and mood stabilisers
Psychotomimetics

ANXIOLYTICS AND HYPNOTICS

Most anxiety-relieving drugs produce sleep in large enough doses, and sleep inducing drugs relieve anxiety when given during waking hours. Thus many of these agents are used for both purposes.

ANXIOLYTICS

These are over widely prescribed: they should not be routinely given for stress-related symptoms, unhappiness, depression, phobic or obsessional conditions. Dependence and tolerance readily develop and therefore they should only be used in the lowest effective doses for the shortest time. The drugs used are:
   benzodiazepines (mainly)
   also: buspirone; chlormezanone; hydroxyzine; meprobamate.

Other types of drug used in the treatment of anxiety
β-blockers
antidepressants

BENZODIAZEPINES

Main actions
1. Anxiolytic (hypnotic in larger doses)
2. Anticonvulsant
3. Muscle relaxant.

Mechanisms of action
Act on specific (BZ) receptors. Potentiation of effects of central
inhibitory transmitter gamma aminobutyric acid.
Muscular relaxation due to inhibition of polysynaptic reflexes in the
spinal cord.
Depression of limbic system more than neocortex and ascending
reticular formation.

Metabolic interrelationships of some benzodiazepines
All of these substances are pharmacologically active anxiolytics
(underlined compounds employed as therapeutic substances).

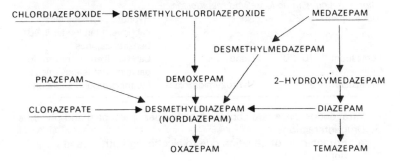

Fig. 10.1

General pharmacokinetic properties
Well absorbed orally. Highly protein bound (over 85%) in plasma.
Volume of distribution typically 1–2 l/kg. Negligible enzyme induction.
Some (e.g. diazepam) have long $t_{1/2}$ others (e.g. lorazepam) have a
shorter $t_{1/2}$ and no active metabolites.

Adverse effects
1. CNS
   a. Sedation, apathy, proneness to motor accidents
   b. Memory impairment
   c. Weakness, ataxia, dysarthria, diplopia
   d. Confusion, intoxication, aggression
   e. Paradoxical excitement and anxiety
   f. Depression (and suicide)
   g. In patients with organic brain disease—prone to produce
      tremulousness, crying, nocturnal and morning confusion,
      agitation
2. Allergic reactions: uncommon
3. Other systems
   a. No clearly defined effects on kidneys, liver and fetus
   b. Mild depression of respiration and blood pressure

Table 10.1 Examples of benzodiazepines

Drug	Elimination $t_{1/2}$ (hours)	Active metabolites	Special features
Longer acting with active metabolites			
Diazepam	20–50	Desmethyldiazepam ($t_{1/2}$ = 100 h)	Used in anxiety as a hynotic and i.v. for profound sedation and status epilepticus
Flurazepam	2	Desalkyflurazepam ($t_{1/2}$ = 200 h)	Hypnotic
Shorter acting with no long-lived metabolites			
Temazepam	5–20	None	Hypnotic; perhaps less hangover than longer lived benzodiazepines
Lorazepam	10–20	None	Can be given i.v. or i.m. for panic or status epilepticus
Midazolam	2	Hydroxymidazolam	i.v. for profound sedation

4. Intravenous diazepam can produce apnoea, local pain and phlebitis
5. Drug interactions:
   a. Potentiation of sedation due to alcohol and other central depressants
   b. Excitement and aggression with alcohol
6. Drug dependence:
   a. Acute withdrawal after 4–8 days: anxiety, insomnia, fits
   b. Chronic anxiety, agoraphobia
   c. Sensory disorders (e.g. covered in cotton wool; headaches; muscle pains; photophobia; hyperacousis; hyperalgesia)
   d. Auditory and visual hallucinations
   e. Depression
   f. Gastrointestinal symptoms
7. Drug overdose: respiratory depression is not usually lethal unless other central depressants are given concurrently or lung disease present.

Clinical uses
1. Hypnotic
2. Anxiolytic
3. Acute panic
4. Premedication in surgery
5. Psychosedative in investigations and operations
6. Anticonvulsant
7. Muscle relaxant in tension states and spasticity.

Flumazenil is an antagonist of the BZ receptor and can reverse the sedative actions of the benzodiazepines.

Buspirone
Has a different mode of action from benzodiazepines and does not prevent benzodiazepine withdrawal state. It takes up to 2 weeks to act. Palpitations, excitement and aggravation of epilepsy can happen.

Chlormezanone
Produces sleepiness and reduces muscle spasm. Also used as a hypnotic, but leaves a hangover the next day.

Hydroxyzine
An H_1 antihistamine used in the short term treatment of anxiety.

Meprobamate
Less effective anxiolytic than benzodiazepines but more dangerous in overdose.

β blockers
Suppress tremor and tachycardia due to anxiety.

Antidepressants
May be effective in chronic anxiety and in phobic and obsessive disorders.

HYPNOTICS
Drugs to induce sleep are greatly over used—the major disadvantages being the rapid production of tolerance and dependence. Withdrawal can be difficult because of insomnia, vivid dreams and anxiety. When used at all they should be prescribed for short periods only.
  Sedative actions usually persist into the following day (hangover). In the elderly, confusion and tendency to falls are produced. The main hypnotics are:
  benzodiazepines
  chlormethiazole
  zopiclone
  promethazine
  barbiturates
  alcohol
  chloral.

Chlormethiazole
Very short $t_{1/2}$ thus less morning confusion in the elderly. Reduces insomnia and proneness to fit during alcohol withdrawal—but used for a week or less, as readily causes dependence.

Zopiclone
Not a benzodiazepine but same mode of action. Causes bitter taste, nausea and hangover.

Promethazine
Sedative antihistamine with anti-itch and anti-nausea actions. Can cause respiratory depression.

Barbiturates
Ultra short acting forms (thiopentone and methohexitone) still used as intravenous anaesthetic. Phenobarbitone used an anticonvulsant. Medium acting forms (e.g. amylobarbitone and pentobarbitone) no longer recommended because of powerful respiratory depression, enzyme induction and rapid dependence.

Alcohol
Not recommended as an hypnotic because of dependence, confusion and hangover. It causes wakefulness and anxiety during the night after its effects have worn off.

Chloral
This is an irritant of the stomach, mouth and skin. It can cause respiratory depression.

NEUROLEPTICS (ANTIPSYCHOTIC DRUGS)

1. Basic action is to reduce dopamine-medicated activity in the brain, (block D_2, non-adenyl cyclase-linked, dopamine receptors)
2. Effective in excited psychotic states (schizophrenia, hypomania, delirium, drug withdrawal syndromes).

MAIN TYPES OF NEUROLEPTICS

Chemical group	Examples
Phenothiazines	
Aliphatic side chains	Chlorpromazine
Piperidine side chains	Thioridazine
Piperazine side chain	Trifluoperazine
	Prochlorperazine
Butyrophenones	Haloperidol
Thioxanthines	Flupenthixol
Diphenylbutylpiperidines	Pimozide
Other structures	Loxapine
	Sulpiride
	Clozapine

Tetrabenzine and reserpine have neuroleptic activity. They act by depletion of neuronal stores of amine transmitters.

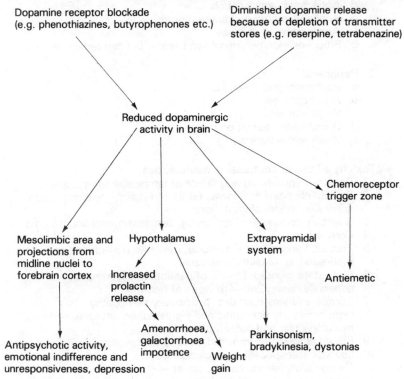

Fig 10.2 Dopamine theory of actions of neuroleptics.

MAIN ACTIONS OF PHENOTHIAZINE NEUROLEPTICS

1. Central
Experimental
- a. Taming of wild animals
- b. Reduction of sham rage in experimental animals
- c. Antagonise amphetamine-induced stereotyped behaviour in animals
- d. Slowing in acquisition of learned responses and acceleration of loss of learned responses in animals

Man
- a. Sedation and reduction in attention span
- b. Reduction in emotional responsiveness (ataractic state)
- c. Hypothalamic inhibition:
    - (i) Reduced sympathetic outflow
    - (ii) Loss of temperature control
    - (iii) Increased prolactin release

d. Antiemetic, antihiccough
e. Antihallucinatory and antipsychotic
f. Aggravation of epilepsy
g. Produces extrapyramidal syndromes, but can reduce chorea

2. **Peripheral**
   a. α adrenoceptor blockade
   b. Anticholinergic
   c. Weak anti 5HT
   d. Quinidine-like action on heart
   e. Weak antihistamine (H_1)

Toxicity of the phenothiazine neuroleptics
1. Postural hypotension and failure of temperature regulation
2. Dry mouth, nasal stuffiness, failure of ejaculation, constipation, urinary retention, blurred vision
3. Sedation, drowsiness, confusion, depression, emotional inertia
4. Convulsions
5. Tremor, Parkinsonism, dystonia, dyskinesia, akathisia (motor restlessness), tardive dyskinesias
6. Cholestatic jaundice (2–4% of patients on chlorpromazine, especially during 2nd–4th week of treatment)
7. Corneal and lens opacities, pigmentary retinopathy
8. Light sensitivity dermatitis and pigmentation, urticaria, oedema, maculopapular and petechial rashes
9. Raised cholesterol, impaired glucose tolerance
10. Leucopenia especially with clozapine
11. Cardiac arrhythmias, cardiac arrest
12. Oligomenorrhoea, amenorrhoea, gynaecomastia, galactorrhoea
13. Malignant syndrome: coma, autonomic disturbances.

Drug interactions with the phenothiazines
1. Anticholinergic effects on gastrointestinal tract affect absorption of paracetamol, levodopa, digoxin, lithium
2. Alcohol potentiates sedation
3. Effects of hypnotics and anxiolytics potentiated
4. Sedative, respiratory depressant and 'cortical' effects of narcotic analgesics potentiated
5. Potentiation of hypotensive drugs
6. Chlorpromazine is moderate enzyme inducer, but also inhibits the metabolism of tricyclic antidepressants.

Clinical uses of phenothiazines
1. Psychiatry:
   a. Schizophrenia
   b. Hypomania
   c. Delirium

    d. Drug withdrawal
    e. Panic attacks
2. α blockade:
    a. Shock
    b. Hypertension-reaction with MAOI
3. Terminal illness
4. Antiemetic, antihiccough, Menière's disease
    a. Surgery:
        (i) Premedication
        (ii) Hypothermic techniques
        (iii) Neuroleptanalgesia.

DEPOT NEUROLEPTICS
e.g. Fluphenazine enanthate
     Flupenthixol decanoate.
General features:
1. Long acting (up to 3 weeks per dose)
2. Injected:
    a. Avoids first pass metabolism
    b. Avoids compliance failure
3. About 30% develop extrapyramidal syndromes.

Chorea
Huntington's chorea: imbalance due to intact nigrostriatal
dopaminergic system with a reduction in GABA producing neurones.
May be improved by reducing dopaminergic activity with neuroleptics
(e.g. tetrabenazine, pimozide, thiopropazate).

Anti-spasticity drugs

Drug	Action	Toxicity
Diazepam	Facilitates $GABA_A$-mediated neuronal inhibition	Sedation
Baclofen	Inhibits release of excitatory neurotransmitters in the cord (stimulates $GABA_B$ receptors)	Sedation, vertigo, nausea, hypertension, fits
Dantrolene	Inhibits depolarisation-induced Ca^{2+} release from sarcoplasmic reticulum	Reduction in muscle power, drowsiness, vertigo, malaise

Table 10.2 Comparison of the more widely used neuroleptics

Drug	Sedation	Anticholinergic	Hypotensive and ∝ adrenergic blocking	Extrapyramidal effects	Special features
Chlorpromazine	+ + +	+ +	+ +	+ +	Can produce sensitivity Cholestatic jaundice
Thioridazine	+ +	+ + +	+ +	+	Most prone to produce retinopathy and cardiac toxicity
Trifluoperazine	+ Can be stimulatory	+	+	+ + +	Powerful antiemetic
Haloperidol	+	+	+	+ + +	Also used as a premed Similar to piperazine neuroleptics
Flupenthixol	+ Can be stimulatory	+ +	+ +	+ +	Similar to chlorpromazine but less sedation and has useful antidepressant and anxiolytic activity
Pimozide	+	±	±	+	Useful in chronic schizophrenia but not effective in acute psychomotor agitation

+ + + = marked   + + = moderate   + = mild   ± = virtually absent

Table 10.3 Drug-induced extrapyramidal syndromes

Syndrome	Mechanism	Causative drugs	Treatment
Parkinsonism: Complete syndrome or single features: tremor, akinesia, rigidity, occulogyric crises.	Blockade of extrapyramidal dopamine receptors	Neuroleptics (methyldopa). Metoclopramide	Anticholinergics (not very effective).
Acute dystonic reactions: Within 48 hours of start of treatment: abrupt onset of retrocollis, torticollis, facial grimacing, dysarthria, laboured breathing, involuntary movements, scoliosis, lordosis, opisthotonus, dystonic gait.	? Increase in transmitter turnover.	Neuroleptics Metoclopramide Levodopa.	i.v. benztropine or diazepam (usually effective).
Akathisia: Motor restlessness after days, weeks or months of treatment.	? Increased sensitivity or overstimulation of dopamine receptors.	Neuroleptics Levodopa.	Reduction in drug dose, benzodiazepines (may improve spontaneously).
Chronic tardive dyskinesias: Oro-facial chewing and sucking movements, accompanied by distal limb chorea and dystonia of trunk. 15% of patients treated with neuroleptics for more than 2 years develop this. Can persist after stopping drug.	? 'Denervation hypersensitivity' of dopamine sensitive neurones.	Neuroleptics. Metoclopramide Domperidone	Condition worsens on stopping neuroleptic.

Anti-tremor agents (excluding Parkinsonism)

Drug	Action	Type of tremor
β blockers	Inhibition of peripheral β_2 receptors control release of acetylcholine at motor end plate	Thyrotoxicosis Anxiety Benign essential
Primidone	Unknown. Probably potentiates GABA	Benign essential and familial
Benzodiazepines	Central potentiation of $GABA_A$	Anxiety

ANTIDEPRESSANT DRUGS

AMINE THEORY OF MOOD

Depression results from a deficiency of transmitter amines (e.g. dopamine, noradrenaline and/or 5-hydroxytryptamine) at certain central synapses.

Some evidence
Reserpine (depletes amine stores) → depression
Neuroleptics (block central amine receptors) → depression
Some depressed patients have been shown to have low
    concentrations of cerebral amines
Monoamine oxidase inhibitors → increase amine levels in the brain
    and are antidepressant
Tricyclics which block uptake$_1$ of amines into presynaptic neuronal
    stores → increased amine concentration in the synaptic cleft and
    are antidepressant.

ANTIDEPRESSANT DRUGS

1. First line: older tricyclics (e.g. amitriptyline)
2. Second line (e.g. mianserin, viloxazine, trazodone)
3. 5-HT uptake blockers (e.g. lofepramine, fluvoxamine)
4. Monoamine oxidase inhibitors (e.g. phenelzine)
5. Thioxanthines (e.g. flupenthixol)
6. Prophylactic agents (e.g. lithium).

GENERAL PROPERTIES OF TRICYCLIC ANTIDEPRESSANTS

Mode of action
1. Block uptake$_1$ of amines
2. Possible increase in amine receptor sensitivity.

General properties
1. Antidepressant in 50–70% of patients after a delay of 1–3 weeks
2. Peripheral anticholinergic effects
3. Peripheral sympathomimetic effects—especially c.v.s.

Pharmacokinetics
1. Good intestinal absorption but significant first pass metabolism
2. High lipid solubility and very large volume of distribution
3. Prolonged $t_{1/2}$
4. High degree of protein binding.

Toxicity
1. Dry mouth, constipation, retention of urine, aggravation of glaucoma
2. Dangerous cardiac effects in overdose, tachycardias and intracardiac blocks. In normal doses: postural hypotension (common), sudden death (very rare)
3. Aggravation of epilepsy.

Drug interactions of tricyclic antidepressants
Monoamine oxidase inhibitors—potentiation of both drugs
Alcohol—sedation
Anticholinergics—potentiated
Anticonvulsants—antagonism
Antihypertensives—clonidine or adrenergic neurone blockers (e.g. guanethidine)—loss of antihypertensive effect
Directly acting sympathomimetic amines—hypertensive effects potentiated

MONOAMINE OXIDASE INHIBITORS (e.g. phenelzine)

General properties
1. Inhibition of mitochondrial monoamine oxidase which results in enlargement of vesicular stores of noradrenaline, 5HT and dopamine within neurones.
2. Reduce the number of β-adrenergic binding sites. Increase sensitivity to agonists at α_1 and 5HT receptors.

Toxicity
Dangerous interactions with foods and drugs of two types:
1. Indirectly acting sympathomimetic agents (e.g. tyramine, amphetamine, dopamine) displace greatly enlarged stores of noradrenaline in brain, peripheral sympathetic nerve endings and adrenal medulla producing hyperthermia, hypertension and cardiac arrhythmias. Can be treated with α and β blockers.

Table 10.4 Some tricyclic antidepressants

Approved names	$t_{1/2}$ (hours)	Inhibition of uptake$_1$ of:		Central sedation	Special uses
		Noradrenaline	5-HT		
Tertiary amines					
Imipramine	4–18	+ +	+ + +	Insomnia, but moderately sedative	1. Phobic anxiety: prevents panic attacks 2. Nocturnal enuresis
Amitriptyline	8–20 (NB: nortriptyline is a metabolite)	+ +	+ + +	Sedating	Most widely used of all tricyclics
Secondary amine					
Protriptyline	54–198	+ + +	+ +	Least sedative of the tricyclics: may be stimulant	Depression with apathy or retarded features

NOTE: Secondary amines mainly inhibit uptake of noradrenaline, are less sedating and less anticholinergic than are tertiary amines.

Table 10.5 Properties of newer antidepressant drugs

Drug	Mode of action	Special features	Toxicity
Mianserin	Presynaptic α blockade causing amine release.	Tetracyclic. Not anticholinergic. Epileptogenic. Does not produce cardiac arrhythmias in overdose.	Sedation. Postural hypotension.
Viloxazine	Inhibition of uptake$_1$ of noradrenaline. Also increases cerebral concentration of noradrenaline, dopamine and 5HT.	Very little anticholinergic activity. Less prone to produce arrhythmias and fits than tricyclics.	Nausea and vomiting common. Headache.
Flupenthixol	Neuroleptic action related to dopamine receptor blockade. Mechanisms of antidepressant action not known.	Neuroleptic antipsychotic. Given orally or by depot injection. Anxiolytic, but not sedating.	Neuroleptic toxicity.
Trazodone	5HT partial agonist; high concentrations block uptake 1 of 5HT.	$t_{1/2}$ = 3–5h. Anxiolytic.	Sedation; slightly anticholinergic; little cardiotoxicity in overdose.
Fluvoxamine	Selective inhibition of 5HT reuptake	Like other selective 5HT uptake blockers, has little anticholinergic and low cardiotoxic activity	Like other 5HT uptake blockers, reduces appetite and causes nausea.

2. Agents whose action is terminated by oxidation, have a more prolonged and profound effect when their oxidising enzymes are inhibited (e.g. pethidine, barbiturates).

Dangerous interactions between foods and monoamine oxidase inhibitors
1. Cheese (tyramine)
2. Broad bean pods (dopamine)
3. Yeast and meat extracts (mixed amines including histamine)
4. Alcoholic beverages—e.g. beer, Chianti (mixed amines produced by fermentation).

Dangerous interactions between drugs and monoamine oxidase inhibitors
1. Sympathomimetic amines, not directly acting, but indirectly acting such as phenylpropanolamine and amphetamine
2. Levodopa and atropinic anti-Parkinsonian drugs
3. Tricyclic antidepressants
4. Narcotic analgesics.

LITHIUM CARBONATE

Uses
1. Prophylactic agent in recurrent affective disorders
2. Treatment of mania

Mode of action
Unknown. Enters neurones via Na^+ channel.
Inhibits Ca^{2+}—and depolarisation—induced release of noradrenaline and dopamine. Enhances release of 5HT in the hippocampus. Inhibits phosphatidyl inositide formation in neurones and therefore reduces responsiveness to cholinergic and α-adrenergic stimuli.

Pharmacokinetics
Well absorbed from intestine. $t_{1/2}$ = 18–20 h, more prolonged in the elderly. No plasma protein binding. Elimination via kidneys—impaired excretion during sodium diuresis. Optimum plasma level 0.4–1.0 mmol/l.

Adverse effects
Ataxia, tremor, diarrhoea, renal impairment, fits—dose-dependent
Goitre with or without hypothyroidism ⎫
Nephrogenic diabetes insipidus ⎪
ECG abnormalities ⎬ dose-independent
Weight gain ⎭

HALLUCINOGENIC DRUGS
1. **Amphetamine derivatives**
   a. Amphetamine sulphate
   b. Dexamphetamine sulphate
   c. Methamphetamine hydrochloride
   d. Dimethoxyamphetamine (methoxymethylamphetamine; STP; DOM)
   e. 3, 4 methylenedioxyamphetamine (MDA)

2. **Indole derivatives**
   a. Mescaline (from peyote cactus—*Lophophora williamsii*)
   b. Psilocybin + psilocin (from mushrooms—*Psilocybe mexicanum* + *Stropharia cubensis*)
   c. d—lysergic acid diethylamide (LSD) (from ergot—*Claviceps purpurea*)
   d. Dimethyltryptamine (DMT)
   e. Harmaline

3. **Anticholinergics**
   a. Atropine
   b. Stramonium

4. **Cannabis preparations**

5. **Miscellaneous substances**
   a. Methylphenidate
   b. Phenmetrazine
   c. Phencyclidine hydrochloride (PCP; constitutent of 'angel dust')
   d. Petrol and other solvents
   e. Amyl nitrite
   f. Morning glory seeds

Lysergic acid diethylamide (LSD)
1. Initial synthesis from ergot alkaloids
2. Some structural resemblances to 5HT; ? increases cerebral 5HT turnover
3. Potent psychotomimetic
4. Produces tolerance rapidly with cross-tolerance to mescaline and psilocybin but not to cannabinoids or dimethyltryptamine
5. No physical dependence
6. Major complications due to catastrophic psychotic reactions, 'flashback' effects, prolonged changes in mood and effect
7. Minor physiological effects: hyperreflexia, mydriasis, muscular incoordination and seizures
8. Drug abuse with LSD common: usually taken orally, occasionally i.v. or smoked with marihuana.

Usual effects of marihuana
1. Euphoria, elation, relaxation
2. Feelings of detachment, clarity, cleverness
3. Decreased concentration span, disturbed thought, poor memory, wish to transmit insight
4. Increased awareness of sensory stimuli
5. Altered concepts of time and space
6. Suggestibility
7. Rapidly changing emotions
8. Altered sexual feelings
9. Increased appetite and thirst, or nausea
10. Dizziness, sleepiness
11. Paraesthesiae, weakness of limbs, sensations of floating, changes in body image
12. Restlessness, ataxia, tremor
13. Dry mouth, tachycardia, urinary frequency, injected conjunctivae
14. Hangover.

Dysphoric intoxication ('bad trip')
1. Anxiety, panic, fear of dying
2. Depression, paranoia
3. Hallucinations
4. Fear of going mad
5. Sensations of nausea and precordial constriction.

Prolonged adverse reactions
1. Confusion, panic, hallucinations, and paranoia may persist for hours or days
2. Hallucinations and effects of marihuana may recur weeks or months after smoking. These are called 'flashbacks'
3. Chronic psychotic conditions, e.g. dementia, depression
4. Chronic physical conditions, e.g. respiratory, ophthalmic, gastrointestinal, dermatological and sleep disturbances
5. Antimotivational syndrome—possibly does not exist per se, but represents underlying mental illness.

ANTICONVULSANT DRUGS

Mode of action
1. Selective blockade of repetitive neuronal discharge at concentrations below those which block conduction of a single impulse.
2. Phenytoin blocks propagation of epileptic electrical discharge, whilst phenobarbitone suppresses excitability of epileptic focus.
3. Sodium valproate, clonazepam, diazepam, nitrazepam and vigabatrin increase effects of central inhibitory transmitter, GABA.

Valproate inhibits decarboxylation of GABA, and vigabatrin irreversibly inhibits GABA transaminase.
4. Phenytoin, primidone and phenobarbitone possibly antagonise the excitatory actions of folate in the brain but their main action is inhibition of picrotoxin receptor (part of the GABA receptor). The result of this type of drug action is thus a more prolonged opening of the chloride channel in the presence of GABA.

DRUG TREATMENT OF VARIOUS FORMS OF EPILEPSY

Type of epilepsy	*Drugs most likely to be successful*
Petit mal absences with a 3 Hz spike and wave pattern in the EEG	Ethosuximide and/or valproate
Hypsarrhythmia with salaam attacks—a form a myoclonic epilepsy in early childhood with generally poor prognosis	Corticotrophin, steroids, clonazepam
Myoclonic and akinetic attacks with a 2 Hz spike and wave pattern on the EEG	Clonazepam, valproate
Tonic—clonic seizures	Carbamazepine, valproate, phenytoin
Partial seizures including psychomotor and psychosensory epilepsy	First line: carbamazepine, valproate, phenytoin. Second line: vigabatrin, phenobarbitone, acetazolamide, clonazepam, primidone, clobazam

NB Treatment is begun using one drug, and if tolerated, this is increased in dosage to its maximum efficacy (guided by blood levels) before adding or substituting another drug.

Pharmacokinetics

Ethosuximide
1. $t_{1/2}$ = 70 h in adults
2. $t_{1/2}$ = 30 h in children
3. Optimum plasma level 40–120 µg/ml
4. Very little plasma protein binding
5. The two main metabolites are inactive.

Clonazepam
1. $t_{1/2}$ = 10–20 h. No active metabolites
2. Poor correlation between blood level and effect
3. Not an inducer.

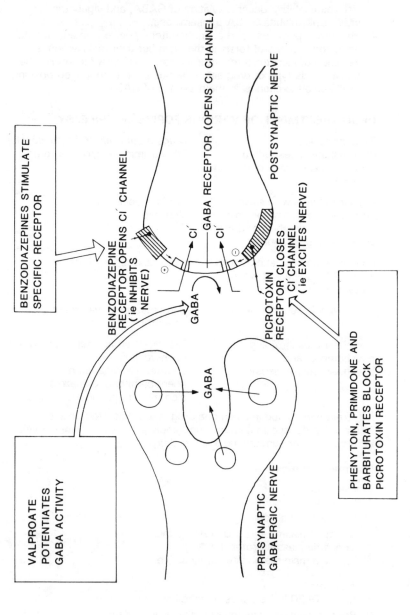

Fig. 10.3 Anticonvulsant drugs and the gamma amino butyric acid (GABA) receptor complex.

Phenytoin
1. Variable intestinal absorption—peak at 2–4h. Very slow absorption from i.m. injection
2. Removed mainly by metabolism to p-hydroxy derivative; 5% excreted unchanged
3. Non-linear (Michaelis–Menten) kinetics, i.e. zero order elimination over the therapeutic range
4. Large genetic variation in rate of metabolism
   a. $t_{1/2}$ depends on plasma level, e.g. on chronic dosage is 140h
   b. 90% protein bound in plasma
   c. Therapeutic range 10–20 µg/ml of plasma
   d. Metabolism impaired by isoniazid
   e. Metabolism accelerated by carbamazepine.

Carbamazepine
1. Enzyme inducer. $t_{1/2}$ of single dose 20–60h, but after chronic therapy becomes 10h
2. Metabolism of warfarin and pill accelerated
3. Main metabolite is carbamazepine-10, 11-epoxide: one-third as active.
4. Therapeutic range 4–12 µg/ml plasma.

Sodium valproate
Completely metabolised; $t_{1/2}$ = 12h Plasma level of 50–100 µg/ml correlates poorly with clinical effect. Not an inducer.

Vigabatrin
Excreted unchanged in urine; $t_{1/2}$ = 5h; not protein bound; not an inducer; lowers blood level of phenytoin.

Phenobarbitone
1. Powerful enzyme inducer
2. First order (linear) kinetics
3. $t_{1/2}$ = 100h in adults
4. $t_{1/2}$ = 40h in children
5. Therapeutic range 15–40 µg/ml.

Primidone
1. Two main metabolites (both of which are anticonvulsant)—phenobarbitone and phenylethylmalonamide (PEMA)
2. Primidone is also anticonvulsant
3. $t_{1/2}$ = 10h (but of metabolite phenobarbitone is 100h).

Toxicity of anticonvulsants

Carbamazepine	Mild ataxia and sedation. Water intoxication and leucopenia. Craniofacial and other defects in fetus when taken in early pregnancy.
Sodium valproate	Mild sedation and gastrointestinal disturbance. Reversible hair loss. Hepatic necrosis (rare). Spina bifida in fetus when taken in early pregnancy.
Phenytoin	Cerebellar signs. Blood dyscrasias. Fetal abnormalities when taken in early pregnancy: Orofacial clefts and congenital heart disease.
Vigabatrin	Sedation. Depression, confusion, psychosis, weight gain.
Phenobarbitone and primidone	Very sedating. Paradoxical excitement. Severe aggravation of epilepsy on rapid withdrawal.

ANTIPARKINSONIAN DRUGS

Parkinsonism
1. Idiopathic (Parkinson's disease)
2. Post encephalitic
3. Toxic (Mn, CO, phenyl tetrahydropyridine)
4. Reversible drug effects (neuroleptics).

The Parkinsonian syndrome
This is due to:
1. *Reduction* in activity of dopaminergic (inhibitory) nigro-striatal pathway terminating in caudate nucleus resulting in diminished transmission at D_2 receptors *or*
2. *Increase* in activity of cholinergic (excitatory) fibres terminating in caudate nucleus.

TREATMENT

1. Withdraw cause (e.g. stop neuroleptic)
2. Block cholinergic activity in caudate by using anticholinergic drugs, e.g. atropine, benztropine; benzhexol
3. Increase dopaminergic activity:
   a. Increase dopamine in caudate nucleus—levodopa, levodopa plus decarboxylase inhibitors
   b. Stimulate dopamine receptors
      (i) Bromocriptine
      (ii) Lysuride
   c. Release of endogenous dopamine
      Amantadine
   d. Block uptake$_1$ of dopamine
      (i) Benztropine
      (ii) Benzhexol

e. Inhibition of monoamine oxidase type B: selegiline. Used with levodopa and decarboxylase inhibitors in late disease, and on its own in early disease to retard progress of the disease.

Levodopa (L-dopa)

Benefits two-thirds of patients with Parkinson's disease. Important limitation to its use is toxicity, particularly:
1. Nausea and vomiting (stimulation of DA receptors in the chemoreceptor trigger zone)
2. Postural hypotension (stimulation of NA receptors in the vasomotor centre)
3. Involuntary movements (dystonic reactions) (stimulation of DA receptors in the caudate nucleus)
4. Psychological disturbances (stimulation of DA receptors in the limbic system)
5. Cardiac arrhythmias (stimulation of β adrenergic receptors in the heart).

Levodopa passes through the blood–brain barrier and is converted to dopamine in the CNS. Peripheral conversion to dopamine (which does not pass through the blood–brain barrier) is inhibited by:

1. Carbidopa ⎫ peripheral dopa
2. Benserazide ⎭ decarboxylase inhibitors

The advantages of combining levodopa with a decarboxylase inhibitor are:
1. 4–5 fold reduction in levodopa dosage
2. Incidence of nausea is reduced
3. Incidence of cardiac arrhythmias is reduced
4. Clinical benefit appears earlier.

ALCOHOL

The most important drug of dependence (5% of adult population in the West are alcohol-dependent).

Pharmacokinetics

Absorbed from mouth, oesophagus, stomach and intestines. Widely distributed in body. 5% excreted in breath and urine unchanged ($V_d = 0.6$ l/kg).

Rate of metabolism obeys Michaelis–Menten kinetics and is approximately 10 ml ethanol/hour.

Acute effects of alcohol
1. *CNS*—decreases in:
   a. Motor coordination
   b. Learning ability

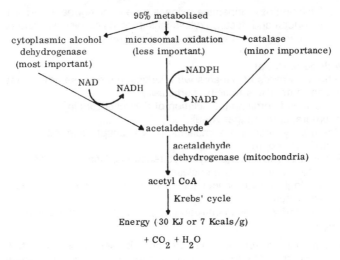

Fig. 10.4

  c. Association formation
  d. Attention span and concentration
  e. Versatility
  f. Judgement, discrimination and reasoning
  In non-drinkers there is a rough correlation between blood levels
  and central effects:
  a.   20 mg/100 ml mild social de-inhibition
  b.   30 mg/100 ml euphoria
  c.   50 mg/100 ml mild uncoordination
  d.   100 mg/100 ml obvious ataxia
  e.   300 mg/100 ml stupor, vomiting
  f.   400 mg/100 ml deep anesthesia
  g.   500 mg/100 ml respiratory depression, death
2. *Circulatory system:* sweating and cutaneous vasodilatation,
   splanchnic vasoconstriction, increased heart rate and raised cardiac
   output. These unpleasant effects are increased in individuals with
   low acetaldehyde dehydrogenase activity (e.g. orientals).
3. *Gastrointestinal system:* dilute alcohol stimulates gastric secretion;
   concentrated alcohol inhibits gastric secretion and causes gastritis.
4. *Metabolism:* Inhibition of ADH secretion, metabolic acidosis due to
   increased excretion of ammonium ions.
5. *Other:* raised plasma triglycerides, hyperuricaemia in those prone
   to gout, hypoglycaemia (due to inhibition of gluconeogenesis by
   NADH).

Chronic effects of alcohol
1. *Gastrointestinal system*
   a. Chronic gastritis and peptic ulcer
   b. Haemorrhage due to
      (i) varices
      (ii) gastritis
      (iii) peptic ulcer
      (iv) Mallory–Weiss syndrome
   c. Acute, sub-acute and chronic pancreatitis
   d. Fatty liver (reversible)
   e. Cirrhosis of the liver (irreversible)
2. *Nervous system*
   a. Vitamin deficiency states
      (i) Peripheral neuropathy
      (ii) Wernicke's encephalopathy
      (iii) Korsakoff's psychosis
   b. Alcohol withdrawal
      (i) Tremor
      (ii) Vomiting
      (iii) Anxiety
      (iv) Delirium tremens
      (v) Convulsions
   c. Direct effects of alcohol on the brain
      (i) Chronic cerebral degeneration
      (ii) Cerebellar degeneration
      (iii) Degeneration of corpus callosum (Marchiafava Bignami syndrome)
      (iv) Central pontine gliosis
      (v) Pathological drunkenness (in patients with pre-existing brain damage)
      (vi) Psychiatric syndromes including auditory hallucinations, paranoia, depression (with ideas of suicide), hysterical fugues
3. *Muscles*
   a. Skeletal myopathy
   b. Cardiomyopathy
4. *Blood*
   a. Leucopenia
   b. Thrombocytopenia
   c. Raised high density lipoprotein.

Drug interactions with alcohol
1. Antabuse-type reaction (flushing, headache, nausea, shock) produced by:
   a. Antabuse
   b. Chlorpropamide and other sulphonylureas
   c. Metronidazole
   d. Procarbazine

    e. Furazolidone
2. Potentiation of central depression due to:
    a. Barbiturates and other hypnotics (including chloral)
    b. Antihistamines
    c. Hyoscine
    d. Antidepressants (e.g. amitriptyline)
    e. Benzodiazepines
    f. Neuroleptics (e.g. chlorpromazine)
    g. Opioids
3. Alcohol is a relatively weak enzyme inducer but may lead to reduction in blood levels of oral anticoagulants and phenytoin
4. Inhibition of metabolism of:
    a. Chloral hydrate
    b. Oral hypoglycaemics
5. Accentuation of hypoglycaemia due to:
    a. Insulin
    b. Sulphonylureas
    c. Biguanides
       by inhibiting hepatic gluconeogenesis
6. Potentiation of aspirin-induced gastritis.

Uses
1. Sterilisation of skin
2. Methanol poisoning
Others not established:
3. General anaesthetic
4. Uterine relaxant
5. Vasodilator after acute limb vessel occlusion.

NICOTINE
1. Stimulation followed by paralysis of autonomic ganglia:
    a. Tachycardia
    b. Bradycardia
    c. Vasoconstriction in the skin and viscera with:
       (i) A rise in diastolic blood pressure
       (ii) Salivation
       (iii) Increased peristalsis
       (iv) Bronchial secretion
2. Stimulation followed by paralysis of cholinergic receptors in the motor end plate: twitching, followed by paralysis of voluntary muscle
3. Stimulation of sensory receptors, e.g. carotid body chemoreceptors:
    a. Reflex increase in respiration rate
    b. Reflex increase in blood pressure
    c. Reflex increase in cardiac output
4. Release of catecholamines from adrenal medulla. Increase in blood glucose and fatty acids

5. Central stimulation:
   a. Wakefulness
   b. Tremor
   c. Fits
   d. Diminished appetite, vomiting
   e. Tachypnoea
   f. Secretion of ADH
   g. Euphoria
6. Dependence: abstinence syndrome.

Smoking
1. Most cigarettes contain 1–4 mg nicotine and cigars 15–40 mg nicotine (NB adult oral toxic dose is 60 mg)
2. Absorption of nicotine by oral mucosa, lungs, gastrointestinal mucosa and skin
3. 90% of nicotine inhaled in smoke is absorbed
4. 80–90% of absorbed nicotine is metabolised
5. Enzyme induction? due to other constituents of cigarette smoke
6. Toxic amblyopia due to cyanide in smoke.

Effects of smoking
1. Increased mortality ratio:
   a. Men under 70 years 2:1
   b. Men over 70 years 1.5:1

Excess of mortality mainly due to ischaemic heart disease especially myocardial infarction. Other causes of illness and death positively related to smoking:
1. Cancers of lung, other parts of respiratory tract, oesophagus, mouth, pharynx, cervix, bladder, rectum, pancreas
2. Premature aging of lungs
3. Chronic bronchitis and emphysema, respiratory TB, pneumonia
4. Pulmonary heart disease
5. Non-syphilitic aortic aneurysm
6. Hernia (because of coughing)
7. Atherosclerotic disease, including ischaemic heart disease, stroke
8. Peptic ulcer
9. Buerger's disease and other peripheral occlusive vascular disease
10. Obstetric problems: premature births, small babies, raised perinatal mortality, children show slower school progress
11. Increased incidence of respiratory infections in children of smoker, due to 'passive smoking', i.e. inhalation of parent's tobacco smoke.

Reduced incidence of:
1. Parkinson's disease
2. Ulcerative colitis
3. Alzheimer's dementia.

11. Drugs affecting the central nervous system II. Analgesics

MINOR ANALGESICS
1. Paracetamol and related drugs
2. Anti-inflammatory analgesics (non steroidal anti-inflammatory drugs (NSAID))
   a. Aspirin and other salicylates
   b. Arylalcanoic acid derivatives— { phenylacetic acid derivatives, e.g. diclofenac phenylpropionic acid derivatives, e.g. ibuprofen
   c. Anthranilic acid derivatives; e.g. fenamates
   d. Pyrazolone compounds, e.g. phenylbutazone and oxyphenbutazone
   e. Indoleacetic acid derivatives, e.g. indomethacin, sulindac.

PARACETAMOL

Actions
Analgesic and antipyretic (inhibits brain prostaglandin synthetase but mechanism of analgesia not understood); not a gastric irritant; no peripheral anti-inflammatory activity.

Pharmacokinetics
Rapid absorption from intestine. Bioavailability and absorption rate increased by metoclopramide and exercise, decreased by carbohydrate and sleep.
1. Plasma $t_{1/2}$ = 75–180 minutes. 25–50% plasma protein bound
2. Urinary excretion
   a. Sulphate 25%
   b. Glucuronide 75%
   c. Unchanged drug 1–40%.

94

In overdose
1. Metabolic capacity of drug is exceeded and $t_{1/2}$ is prolonged to 4–12 h or more (above 4 hours liver damage occurs)
2. A reactive metabolite is formed which is hepatotoxic.

Toxicity
1. Rashes (uncommon)
2. Blood dyscrasias (uncommon)
3. Liver damage in overdose
4. Possible nephrotoxicity following high doses for prolonged periods.

Benorylate
Acetylsalicylic ester of paracetamol which is hydrolysed to aspirin and paracetamol by esterases in the plasma and liver. As the ester is absorbed intact, the gastric irritant properties of the salicylate are reduced. Benorylate is thus a prodrug of paracetamol and salicylate.

NON-STEROIDAL ANTI-INFLAMMATORY DRUGS (NSAID)

The NSAID share many properties because of their identical mode of action which is inhibition of cylooxygenase in the eicosanoid synthetic pathway. The result of this (Fig. 11.1) is blockade of synthesis of thromboxanes, prostaglandins and prostacyclin.

Therapeutic actions
1. Inhibition of pain and inflammation is due to reduced synthesis of prostaglandins. These stimulate pain fibres, potentiate pain due to other stimuli (e.g. kinins) and mediate vascular and exudative responses to injury
2. Antipyretic actions due to blockade of formation of PGE in the hypothalamus in response to pyrogens
3. Antithrombotic (and hence anti-atheroma) actions due to inhibition of thromboxane synthesis in platelets. Low dose of aspirin and other NSAID do not cause prolonged blockade of the formation of the natural anti-aggregant of platelets, prostacyclin, by the vascular endothelium.

Toxic effects
1. Peptic ulceration is caused and aggravated by NSAID because prostaglandins reduce gastric acid secretion, increase mucus secretion, vasodilate submucosa and increase cell turnover in the alimentary mucosa. A synthetic prostaglandin, misoprostol, can heal existing peptic ulcers and prevent NSAID-induced gastric ulceration.
2. Allergic reactions and worsening of asthma are probably related to arachidonic acid being preferentially metabolised into the

lipoxygenase pathway with the increased formation of leukotrienes which play a role in atopic disease.
3. NSAID can delay the onset of labour in pregnant women. This is presumably due to inhibition of prostaglandin synthesis. The onset of labour can be hastened or abortion induced by administration of prostaglandins such as $PGF_{2\alpha}$ and dinoprostone.
4. NSAID cause renal changes. High doses taken over a prolonged period are associated with progressive decline in renal function even after stopping the drug (analgesic nephropathy). The initial renal lesion is papillary necrosis. The disease may be due to loss of the natural vasodilator action of prostaglandins. A late consequence of analgesic nephropathy is an increased risk of carcinoma of the renal pelvis.
5. NSAID-related liver damage may be due to a similar mechanism as in analgesic nephropathy.
6. Animal experiments have demonstrated that NSAID can close the ductus arteriosus of the foetus. Aspirin and similar drugs have been used to stimulate closure of a patent ductus in newborn infants.

ASPIRIN (ACETYLSALICYLIC ACID)

Pharmacokinetics
Absorbed via stomach and intestine. Considerable hepatic first pass metabolism. $t_{1/2}$ = 20–30 minutes for acetylsalicylic acid. Principal active substance in circulation is salicylate (although acetylsalicylate is more active). Renal excretion enhanced by alkalinisation of urine.
    Elimination of salicylate obeys overall non-linear kinetics, i.e. the $t_{1/2}$ is dose-dependent.
    Salicylurate formation via a mitochondrial enzyme (unusual) and is easily saturated thus composition of total metabolic products varies with dose and plasma level may rapidly increase once Michaelis–Menten processes are saturated.

Toxicity
1. Dyspepsia—common
   Gastritis and mucosal erosion—very common
   Severe haemorrhage—uncommon
   Possibly due to precipitation of protective glycoprotein as well as removal of the anti-ulcer effects of PGE_2 and $PGF_{2\alpha}$
2. Allergy and non-allergic asthma and urticaria
3. Dose-dependent salicylism (tinnitus, deafness, nausea, abdominal pain)
4. Overdose can initially produce a respiratory alkalosis. In severe poisoning this is followed by metabolic acidosis
5. Gout (low doses of salicylate cause urate retention; large doses are uricosuric)

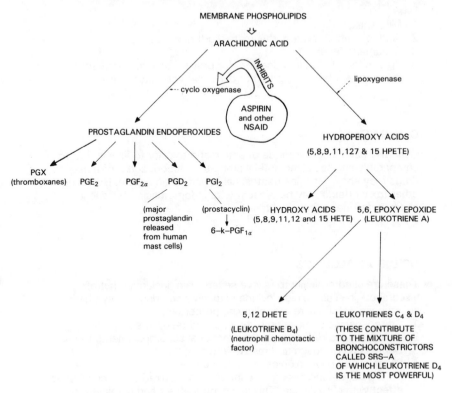

Fig. 11.1 Eicosanoid synthesis and site of action of aspirin and other NSAID.

6. Potentiation of effects of hypoglycaemic agents, anticoagulants and gastric irritants
7. Hepatotoxicity and nephrotoxicity
8. Water retention
9. Reye's syndrome (liver and brain damage) in young children.

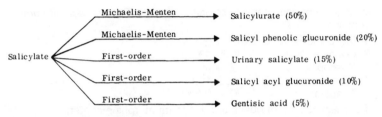

Fig. 11.2 Metabolism of aspirin.

Uses
1. Mild analgesic
2. Anti-inflammatory, e.g. rheumatoid arthritis
3. Rheumatic fever
4. Prevention of platelet adhesion: for prevention and treatment of myocardial infarction and other occlusive vascular disease.

OTHER NSAID

Generally have a similar mode of action and toxicity to aspirin, but for comparable analgesic and anti-inflammatory action, some of these drugs may show less gastrointestinal toxicity than aspirin. However, other toxic effects may be present (e.g. indomethacin—headache; phenylbutazone—agranulocytosis).

OPIOID ANALGESICS

These are used clinically to relieve severe pain, including that of visceral origin. The opioids include naturally occurring and synthetic substances which share the following properties:
1. Stereospecific stimulation of brain opioid receptors
2. Analgesia and reduction of the emotional accompaniments to pain
3. Depression of cough and respiration
4. Physical and psychological dependence
5. Tolerance, i.e. increasing amount of drug required to produce same effect with chronic use. This is a central effect and unrelated to enzyme induction and increased drug metabolism
6. Constipation
7. Vomiting
8. Antagonism of actions by opioid antagonists such as naloxone.

OPIUM

Dried juice of seed capsule of oriental poppy (*Papaver somniferum*) contains:
1. Morphine   (9–17%)
2. Codeine   (0.5–4%)
3. Noscapine   (2–9%)
4. Papaverine   (0.5–1%)
5. Thebaine   (0.1–0.8%).
The main actions of opium are due to its morphine content.

Table 11.1 Mild analgesics with anti-inflammatory action

Drug	Pharmacokinetics	Actions (all inhibit prostaglandin synthetase)	Toxicity
DICLOFENAC	$t_{1/2}$ = 1–2h. Available as slow release form	Powerful analgesic and anti-inflammatory	Rashes and gastrointestinal irritation
IBUPROFEN	$t_{1/2}$ = 2 h	Weak anti-inflammatory	Rashes and gastrointestinal irritation relatively uncommon
MEFENAMIC ACID	Slow absorption from intestine. Peak plasma levels at 2–3h. 99% bound to plasma proteins.	Weak anti-inflammatory	Diarrhoea. Rarely: bone marrow depression, haemolytic anaemia
PHENYLBUTAZONE (and OXYPHENBUTAZONE)	Extensive liver metabolism to drug glucuronide and to *oxyphenbutazone* (which has same properties as phenylbutazone). $t_{1/2}$ = 58–86h	Powerful anti-inflammatory and antipyretic aspirin	Commonly (10–20%) produces rashes. Dyspepsia and irritation of peptic ulcers. Salt and water retention. Drug interactions due to displacement from protein binding. Uncommon: bone marrow depression, hepatitis, severe gastrointestinal haemorrhage. Withdrawn from common use because of toxicity

(contd)

Table 11.1 (contd)

Drug	Pharmacokinetics	Actions (all inhibit prostaglandin synthetase)	Toxicity
INDOMETHACIN	Well absorbed following oral or rectal administration. 90% bound to plasma proteins. Volume of distribution 0.5–0.8 l/kg. Extensive metabolism, with enterohepatic circulation of indomethacin and metabolites. Twice daily dosage	Powerful anti-inflammatory	Commonly (25%) produces headache. Light headedness, confusion, gastric irritation. Salt and water retention. Less prone to produce gastric bleeding than phenylbutazone.
NAPROXEN	Twice daily dosage	One of the most useful analgesics Powerful anti-inflammatory	Relative low incidence of NSAID toxicity
PIROXICAN	High protein binding. Once daily dosage	Powerful anti-inflammatory	Upper gastrointestinal irritation

Also: fenoprofen, tiaprofenic acid, azapropazone, etodolac, nabumetone, sulindac and tenoxicam may prove to be similar to naproxen.

Table 11.2 Additional drugs used in rheumatoid arthritis

Drug	Kinetics	Actions	Toxicity
GOLD SALTS	Given by i.m. injection or orally (less well absorbed). Bound to plasma proteins. Concentrated in inflamed areas. Very slow excretion.	Inhibits PG synthesis. Inhibits lysosomal enzymes. Binds to immunoglobulin and complement. Possibly modifies connective tissue metabolism.	Rashes. Renal damage. Blood dyscrasias. Stomatitis. Diarrhoea with oral gold.
PENICILLAMINE (β dimethylcysteine)	Well absorbed from intestine. Tight binding to plasma proteins. Slow excretion.	Dissociates macroglobulins. Inhibits release of lysosomal enzymes. Chelation of immune complexes.	Nausea, vomiting. Abdominal discomfort. Rashes. Bone marrow depression. Renal damage. Mammary hyperplasia. Haemolytic anaemia. Mucous membrane ulceration. SLE. Myasthenic syndrome.
CHLOROQUINE	Well absorbed from gut; concentrated in tissues; $t_{1/2}$ 3–7 days.	Not analgesic or anti-inflammatory. Stabilises lysosomal membranes.	Retinal injury
CORTICOSTEROIDS	See page 167	See pages 68 and 169	See page 169
SULPHASALAZINE	Releases sulphapyridine + 5 aminosalicyclate (5AS)	5AS scavenges toxic oxygen radicals from leucoytes	Sulphonamide toxicity
METHOTREXATE	Well absorbed orally and given at low dose once per week.	Inhibits folate metabolism.	Myleosuppression. GI intolerence and oral ulceration. Shock lung.

Opioid receptors (see also Ch. 6)

Four receptor types:

μ Mainly supraspinal analgesia, euphoria, sedation, respiratory depression and dependence

κ Spinal analgesia, miosis, weakly sedating. Dysphoria

σ Dysphoria and hallucinations

δ Actions not understood—perhaps peripheral.

Distribution of opioid receptors:

Highest	Amygdala (limbic system)
	Periaqueductal grey matter (midbrain)
	Hypothalamus
Less	Medial thalamic nuclei
	Head of caudate (extrapyramidal system)
	Spinal cord

met^5-encephalin ⎫
leu^5-encephalin ⎬ Found in corpus striatum, thalamus, substantia
α-endorphin ⎭ gelatinosa of cord

β-endorphin   Stored in pituitary; also in hypothalamus
γ-endorphin   Highest in spinal cord
Dynorphin

β-endorphin and encephalins bind to δ receptors but also have actions on μ receptors. Dynorphin acts on κ and μ receptors.

   The analgesia produced by electrical stimulation of the periventricular and periaqueductal grey matter, by acupuncture and by placebos may be abolished by the narcotic antagonist naloxone. Thus these forms of analgesia may be mediated by the release of endogenous morphine-like substances.

   The neural action of the endorphins is inhibitory (but the hippocampus is excited due to the inhibition of inhibitory influences).

Structures

β-lipotrophin (β-LPH) consists of 91 amino acids (no opioid activity)
met^5-encephalin = 61–65 amino acids of β-LPH
α-endorphin   = 61–76 amino acids of β-LPH
γ-endorphin   = 61–77 amino acids of β-LPH
β-endorphin   = 61–91 is C-fragment amino acids
                  of β-LPH
β-MSH   = 41–58 amino acids of β-LPH
β-LPH and ACTH are part of a larger protein (pro-opiocortin = '31 K') synthesized in the hypothalamus.

Clinically used opioids

Although many opioids are currently in use, they can be classified into three main groups according to their actions on the opioid receptors. The following are examples of agonists, antagonists and partial agonists.

Drug	Receptor		
	μ	κ	σ
Morphine	Agonist	Agonist	—
Naloxone	Antagonist	Antagonist	—
Pentazocine	Weak antagonist	Agonist	Agonist
Buprenorphine	Partial agonist	—	—

μ-RECEPTOR AGONISTS

Actions of morphine

Central
1. Analgesia—particularly prolonged pain; reduction in anxiety and agitation produced by pain. Euphoria accompanies relief from pain
2. Drowsiness and sleep. Initial excitement. Coma in large doses
3. Reduction of sensitivity of respiratory centre to CO_2. Shallow and slow respiration. Cough suppression
4. Vomiting due to stimulation of chemoreceptor trigger zone
5. Pupillary constriction due to stimulation of parasympathetic IIIrd cranial nerve nucleus
6. Hypotension and reduced cardiac output partly due to reduced hypothalamic sympathetic outflow
7. Increased release of ADH. Reduced release of ACTH, FSH and LH.

Peripheral
1. Constipation—partly due to stimulation of cholinergic activity in gut wall ganglia which results in smooth muscle spasm
2. Contraction of smooth muscle in sphincter of Oddi and ureters due to same mechanism. Increases in blood amylase and lipase due to pancreatic stasis
3. Histamine release produces bronchospasm, flushing and arteriolar dilatation.
4. Lowered sympathetic discharge and direct arteriolar dilation results in lowered cardiac output and a fall in blood pressure.

Similar μ receptor agonists include pethidine, codeine and fentanyl. Diamorphine (heroin) is converted to morphine in the brain.

OPIOID ANTAGONISTS

Naloxone
A pure antagonist with no partial agonist activity. It is given by injection to reverse the actions of morphine and similar drugs.

Pentazocine
Has mixed antagonist and agonist actions. Even though it is an
analgesic (κ agonist), it can cause withdrawal symptoms and signs in
addicts (μ antagonist) and produce dysphoria and hallucinations (σ
agonist).

PARTIAL AGONISTS

Buprenorphine
A useful analgesic, but because it is a partial agonist of μ receptors, it
can cause withdrawal, and even pain, in addicts.
Meptazinol
Similar, and like buprenorphine, can cause nausea and vomiting.

Production of uric acid

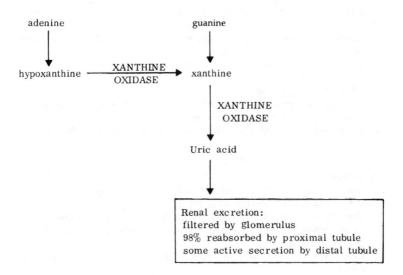

Fig. 11.3

Drugs used in gout
1. Prevention of synthesis of uric acid

Drug	ALLOPURINOL (Zyloric)
Mode of action	Blocks xanthine oxidase
Pharmacokinetics	Well absorbed from intestine
	Plasma $t_{1/2}$ = 3 h
	Metabolised to oxypurinol which is itself a weak xanthine oxidase inhibitor

Toxicity	Rashes Theoretical risk of xanthine stones Block in breakdown of 6-mercaptopurine, azathioprine (dangerous combination) and oral anticoagulants

2. *Uricosuric agents — if allopurinol cannot be used.*

Probenecid
Sulphinpyrazone
Large doses of salicylates (small doses impair urate excretion)

Main drugs used as uricosuric agents

Drug	PROBENECID (Benemid)
Mode of action	Blocks reuptake of uric acid by proximal renal tubule
Pharmacokinetics	*Plasma* $t_{1/2}$ = *8 h*
Toxicity	Rashes, GI upset Nephrotic syndrome (rare)
Other uses	Used to block excretion of penicillin
Drug	SULPHINPYRAZONE (Anturan)
Mode of action	Blocks reuptake of uric acid by proximal renal tubule
Pharmacokinetics	*Plasma* $t_{1/2}$ = *8h*
Toxicity	Rashes, GI upset
Other uses	Reduces risk of myocardial infarction

3. *Acute gout—treatment of acute attack*

NSAID (e.g. indomethacin; naproxen; piroxicam; sulindac)
Glucocorticoids
Colchicine

Drug	COLCHICINE
Mode of action	Binds to microtubular protein and inhibits leucocyte migration and this reduces acute inflammatory reaction.
Pharmacokinetics	Rapidly absorbed from intestine Plasma $t_{1/2}$ = 30 min Partly metabolised and partly excreted in bile. Undergoes an enterohepatic cirulation
Toxicity	Diarrhoea Vomiting

12. Drugs affecting the central nervous system III. Anaesthetics. Also local anaesthetics and neuromuscular blocking drugs

GENERAL ANAESTHESIA

This is a state of unconsciousness in which the subject is not rousable by external stimuli.

Neuronal effects
1. No change in resting potential
2. Anaesthetics produce a rise in threshold of action potential and an inhibition of the rapid increase in sodium permeability. Thus action potentials are inhibited
3. Inhibition of synaptic transmission at excitatory junctions.

Theories of anaesthesia
1. Overton-Meyer: anaesthetic potency varies with fat solubility. Thus equieffective concentrations of anaesthetics multiplied by their fat solubilities gives a constant.
2. Anaesthetics appear to concentrate in hydrophobic regions of cell membranes, causing the membrane to swell and altering the crystalline structure of the membrane. This presumably reduces the ability of the sodium channels to open rapidly.

    General anaesthesia can be reversed by subjecting anaesthetised animals to high enough pressures to reverse membrane swelling.

    Even though general anaesthetics have a wide range of molecular structures, there may be a membrane target of critical size presumably in the hydrophobic portions of protein or phospholipid.
3. Pauling proposed that gaseous anaesthetics might order water structure in the neighbourhood of membranes by forming stable hydrate crystals ('clathrates') which alter membrane function, in particular ionic channels.

Anaesthesia for surgery
This has 3 components:
1. Hypnosis
2. Analgesia
3. Muscular relaxation.
May use different agents to achieve each of these aims separately.

GENERAL ANAESTHETICS

Oil : water and oil : gas partition coefficients determine potency.

Inhalational
1. Halogenated hydrocarbons
    Halothane
    Enflurane and isoflurane
    Trichlorethylene ⎫
    Ethyl chloride   ⎬ almost completely obsolete as general
    Chloroform   ⎭ anaesthetics in the UK
2. Non-halogenated agents
    Nitrous oxide
    Cyclopropane
    Ether

Intravenous
Barbiturates ⎰ Sodium thiopentone
             ⎱ Methohexitone
Etomidate
Propofol
Ketamine

INHALED ANAESTHETICS
1. Onset and offset of action depend on how quickly blood level follows alveolar concentration
2. Main route into and out of the body is via the lungs. Metabolic degradation is usually insignificant during action.

Thus:
Blood : gas partition coefficient determines rate of induction and recovery. Low ratio gives faster induction and recovery; both processes speeded up by rapid alveolar ventilation rate.

Blood flow to the brain is high and the blood brain barrier is very permeable to anaesthetics, thus there is rapid equilibrium between brain concentration and arterial blood concentration. Anaesthetics which dissolve readily in fat have a prolonged recovery phase because of slow release of the drug from adipose tissue (and other cells) back into the blood.

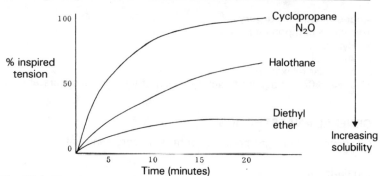

Fig. 12.1 Time for induction varies with solubility of the anaesthetic in blood.

Thus in order to achieve rapid induction with highly soluble anaesthetics it is necessary to administer a concentration in excess of the maintenance concentration.

Halothane

A non-explosive, non-irritant, inhalational anaesthetic. It produces respiratory and cardiovascular depression and can inhibit uterine contractions. Like other halogenated hydrocarbons it can cause liver damage and cardiac dysrhythmias. However the former is rare and the latter uncommon with halothane. Repeated administration increases the risk of liver damage. Metabolites (bromide and trifluroacetic acid) are toxic. It is widely used for induction and maintenance of anaesthesia in major surgery with oxygen, nitrous oxide and muscle relaxants.

Induction and recovery are rapid because of relatively low solubility in blood.

Enflurane

Similar to halothane but is not hepatotoxic and is therefore used instead of halothane when repeated anaesthetics have to be given. Because of lower fat solubility than halothane, it is less potent. Respiratory and myocardial depression are produced, but ventricular dysrhythmias are uncommon.

Very little is metabolised (cf halothane, 30% metabolised).

Isoflurane

An isomer of enflurane. Potency is between that of halothane and enflurane. Even less is metabolised than enflurane. There is little risk of organ toxicity and ventricular dysrhythmics. Muscle relaxation is produced.

Nitrous oxide

Mainly used for its analgesic properties and is widely given in subanaesthetic doses with other anaesthetics in general anaesthesia and on its own for pain management.

Muscle relaxation is not produced. It is not hepatotoxic or cariotoxic, but exposure for long periods can cause anaemia due to interference with vitamin B12 utilisation.
Nitrous oxide (like oxygen) supports combustion.

Cyclopropane
A potent anaesthetic gas. Muscular relaxation is produced. Although recovery is rapid, cyclopropane is not now widely used because of postoperative restlessness and vomiting and because it is explosive.

Ether
Only used nowadays on a named patient basis. The vapour is inflammable and explosive. Ether is irritating to the respiratory mucosa.

INTRAVENOUS ANAESTHETICS
These are usually used as induction agents, but can be used alone for short anaesthetics.
Induction is rapid, often one arm–brain circulation time. Apnoea and hypotension are frequent.

Thiopentone
A barbiturate which is the most widely used induction agent.
Recovery is rapid due to redistribution into muscle, glands and fat after leaving the brain (Fig. 12.2).

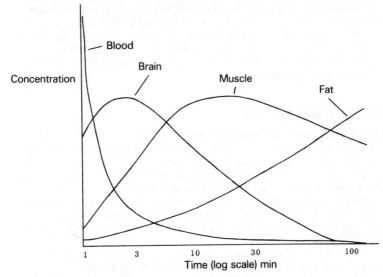

Fig. 12.2 Tissue distribution of thiopentone following intravenous administration.

Metabolism is slow and the drug remains in the body for over 24 hours. The solution is strongly alkaline, and accidental administration into an artery or extravascular tissues is a disaster because of tissue necrosis and possible loss of a limb.

Methohexitone
Similar to thiopentone, but less irritant to the tissue. Although induction may be less smooth, it has an even shorter duration of action than thiopentone. Termination of action is mainly due to tissue redistribution.

Etomidate
Similar to thiopentone but there is a wider margin between the anaesthetic dose and the dose which causes respiratory and cardiovascular depression. Repeated doses suppress adrenal cortical function. It is rapidly metabolised.

Propofol
Widely used in procedures in which the patient returns home the same day because recovery is rapid without hangover. Excitement, fits and local pain may accompany induction.

Ketamine
Used as a general anaesthetic and basal anaesthetic, i.e. it is used in subanaesthetic doses to produce sedation and analgesia. Muscular tone is increased and the blood pressure may be raised.

Hallucinations and other psychological changes are frequent during recovery. Ketamine resembles the hallucinogen phencyclidine structurally and pharmacologically, which is presumably the reason for its psychotic-like toxicity.

LOCAL ANAESTHETICS

Local anaesthetics are applied to mucous membranes or injected into the skin or other tissues to produce analgesia. They act by causing reversible block in conduction along nerve fibres. Their cellular action is to block the initiation and propagation of action potentials in axons by preventing the voltage-dependent opening of sodium channels, which is the basis of axonal transmission of waves of depolarisation. The drug molecule enters the plasma membrane and alters its structure to impede the changes in membrane protein which open the ion channel.

The unionised form of local anaesthetic penetrates the axonal sheath but acts in the cell membrane in its charged form.

Absorbed local anaesthetic can affect the CNS (causing excitement and fits) and the CVS (myocardial depression and vasodilation).

Lignocaine
The most widely used local anaesthetic and can be applied topically or injected. It is often injected with a vasoconstrictor (adrenaline) to prolong its action (up to about $1\frac{1}{2}$ hours).

Bupivacaine
Much longer acting (up to 8 hours) but has a slow onset of action.

Prilocaine
Has low toxicity, and is similar to lignocaine. It is available with a peptide vasoconstrictor, felypressin, which has no direct action on the heart.

Amethocaine and benzocaine
Used for surface anaesthetics.

Procaine
Now seldom used because of its short action. It is ineffective topically.

Cocaine
Still occasionally used for surface anaesthesia, but is never injected because of its toxicity (hypertension, cardiac arrhythmias and CNS stimulation). It is a powerful vasoconstrictor because it blocks uptake 1 of noradrenaline.

MUSCLE RELAXANTS

These cause reversible muscle paralysis. There are two groups —non-depolarising and depolarising.

NON-DEPOLARISING

These are competetive blockers of the nicotinic cholinergic receptor at the motor end plate. Action terminated by anticholinesterases such as edrophonium or neostigmine.

Atracurium
Widely used because its elimination does not depend on enzyme action. It can thus be used in liver and kidney failure. Duration of action is 15–25 minutes. Histamine release may be stimulated.

Vecuronium
Also widely used because of its low toxicity, histamine not being liberated. Duration of action is 20–30 minutes.

Pancuronium
Has no ganglion block action and thus does not lower the blood pressure.

Tubocurarine
Causes histamine release and a fall in blood pressure.

Gallamine
Has a shorter action than other members of the group but causes tachycardia.

Alcuronium
Similar to tubocurarine.

DEPOLARISING (confusingly called 'non-competitive blockers')

These prevent the motor end plate cholinergic receptors responding to acetylcholine by maintaining it in a constant state of depolarisation. Anticholinesterases do not reverse their action.

Suxamethonium
Initially causes fine muscular contractions (fasciculation). Short duration of action — 5 min.

Decamethonium halides
Uncommonly used.

In practice, after the initial phase of depolarisation the drugs of this group produce a curare-like response.

All muscle relaxants are highly charged and do not pass through cell membranes. They are thus administered by intravenous injection.

Uses
1. Muscular relaxation during operations under general anaesthesia
2. Tracheal intubation
3. Facilitation of assisted ventilation
4. Prevention of coughing and laryngospasm during operations.

PREMEDICATION FOR ANAESTHESIA

Purpose
1. Allay anxiety
2. Facilitate induction of anaesthesia
3. Reduce risks of anaesthesia
4. Analgesia
5. Antiemetic.

Premedication agents
1. Anxiolytic agents
2. Narcotic analgesics (opioids)
3. Anticholinergies.

1. Anxiolytic agents
Benzodiazepines (e.g. diazepam)
Antihistamines (H$_1$) (e.g. promethazine) ⎫
Neuroleptics (e.g. chlorpromazine)   ⎬ also antiemetic
Hyoscine.   ⎭

Allay anxiety
Lower levels of circulating catecholamines and thus reduce chance of
    anaesthetic-induced cardiac arrhythmias
Reduce phase of excitement during induction
Reduce postoperative delirium
Some (e.g. hyoscine, promethazine, chlorpromazine) reduce induction
    and postoperative vomiting
Accelerate induction
Reduce amount of anesthetic required
Amnesia for induction (especially benzodiazepines).

2. Narcotic analgesics (e.g. morphine, fentanyl)
Allay anxiety
Reduce pain of surgical illness and antagonise pain-induced shock
Analgesic action allows intubation and operation to be performed with
    less general anaesthetic
Reduce postoperative restlessness due to pain.

3. Anticholinergics (e.g. atropine, hyoscine)
Reduce bronchial, salivary and gastric secretions and thus diminish
    chance of bronchial plugging, aspiration pneumonia and pulmonary
    collapse
Reduce chance of vagal inhibition of heart.

13. Drugs affecting the cardiovascular system

AUTONOMIC CONTROL OF THE HEART AND VESSELS

SYMPATHETIC SYSTEM

Sympathetic nerves—Neurotransmitter is noradrenaline.
Adrenal medulla—Secretions are adrenaline and noradrenaline.

Table 13.1   Effects of sympathetic activity on cardiovascular system

Target organ	Receptor type	Effect of stimulation
Heart	β_1	Increased heart rate
	β_1	Accelerated a–v conduction
	β_1	Increased myocardial excitability
	β_1	Increased contractility
Blood vessels		
Coronary	β_2	Vasodilation
Striated muscle	β_2	Vasodilation
Skin	α	Vasoconstriction
Visceral (including renal)	α	Vasoconstriction

Some vasoconstrictor α receptors also present in myocardial and skeletal muscle arterioles. In vivo of doubtful importance.

PARASYMPATHETIC SYSTEM

Parasympathetic—innervates only nodal and atrial tissue (branches of vagus). Neurotransmitter is acetylcholine.

Effects of parasympathetic activity on the heart
Slows rate of discharge of pacemaker cells, reduces duration of action potential in atrium which results in weak atrial contraction, increases atrioventricular conduction time.

114

PERIPHERAL DOPAMINERGIC SYSTEM

Dopamine—released from dopaminergic fibres, stimulates peripheral dopamine receptors and also stimulates α and β adrenoceptors.
Stimulates cardiac contractility.
Vasodilation (including renal vessels).

Table 13.2 Cardiovascular receptors stimulated by catecholamines

Drug	Receptors			
	α	β_1	β_2	Dopamine
Adrenaline	+ + +	+ +	+	0
Noradrenaline	+ + + +	+ +	+	0
Isoprenaline	0	+ + + +	+ + + +	0
Salbutamol	0	+	+ + + +	0
Dopamine	+ +	+ +	0	+ +
Dobutamine	0	+ +	±	0
Dopexamine	0	0	+ +	+ +
Xamoterol	0	partial agonist	0	0

β-ADRENOCEPTOR BLOCKERS

Block β_1 and β_2 receptors competitively. Cardioselective (β_1) blockers have relatively less action on β_2 receptors in bronchi and peripheral vessels.

Effects of β blockers

CVS	Reduction of exercise- and anxiety-induced tachycardia
	Reduced excitability of myocardium
	Reduction in blood pressure (often delayed)
	Reduced renin release from kidneys
Peripheral nervous system	Reduction of tremor (e.g. due to anxiety)

Toxicity

CVS	Poor exercise tolerance
	Precipitation of heart failure
	Bradycardia and heart block
	Aggravation of intermittent claudication and Raynaud's phenomenon
RS	Bronchospasm in asthmatics
CNS (not all penetrate)	Nightmares, sleep disturbances
	Lack of energy, depression (uncommon)
Metabolic	Potentiation of the action of hypoglycaemic drugs
Others	Impotence
	Diarrhoea
	Muscle cramps

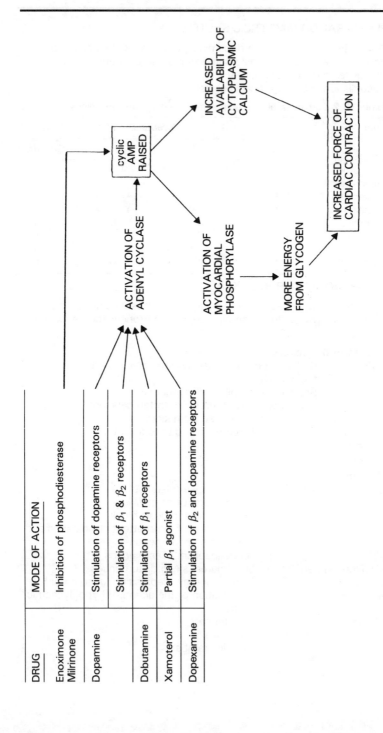

Fig. 13.1 Non-glycoside positive inotropes.

Uses of β blockers
Angina pectoris
Hypertension
Cardiac arrhythmias
Protection against myocardial re-infarction
Others, e.g. migraine, thyrotoxicosis.

POSITIVE INOTROPES

Cardiac glycosides (e.g. digoxin)
Phosphodiesterase inhibitors (enoximone; milrinone)
Sympathomimetics (adrenaline, isoprenaline, dobutamine, dopamine, xamoterol, dopexamine)

These drugs increase the force of contraction of the myocardium. Surprisingly and disappointingly they do not usually have a long-term benefit in cardiac failure. Although digoxin is useful in the treatment of rapid supraventricular arrhythmias, it produces only a small benefit in cardiac failure with a normal rhythm (particularly compared with the effects of diuretics and vasodilators).

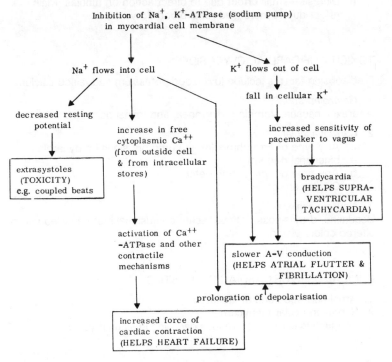

Fig. 13.2 Mode of action of cardiac glycosides.

CARDIAC GLYCOSIDES

Cardiac glycosides = sterol lactone + sugar
(Lactone = aglycone: this has some intrinsic activity, sugar
determines solubility of glycoside but has no pharmacological activity.)

ACTIONS OF CARDIAC GLYCOSIDES

1. *Heart*
    a. Increases force of cardiac contraction
    b. Slows heart rate due to:
        (i) Reduction in compensatory tachycardia due to heart failure
        (ii) Increased sensitivity of sinus node to vagus and increased vagal activity
        (iii) Depression of sinus node discharge
        (iv) Partial a-v block slows heart in artrial fibrillation and flutter
2. *Others*
    a. Peripheral vasoconstriction—not usually important
    b. Diuresis—small effect due to direct action on tubules. Main effect due to increased renal blood flow.

TOXICITY OF CARDIAC GLYCOSIDES

Predisposing factors include low blood potassium and raised calcium.

1. *Gastrointestinal*
Anorexia, nausea, vomiting, diarrhoea, abdominal pain.

2. *Cardiovascular*
    a. Any type of arrhythmia (most common: sinus bradycardia, bigeminal rhythm)
    b. Any type of conduction defect
    c. Cardiac arrest

3. *Neurological*
Headache, drowsiness, fatigue, acute confusional state, blurred vision, altered colour vision.

CLINICAL USES OF CARDIAC GLYCOSIDES

1. Atrial fibrillation and atrial flutter
2. Supraventricular tachycardia
3. Congestive cardiac failure (use declining in sinus rhythm)

Table 13.3 Properties of som β-adrenergic blocking drugs

	PROPRANOLOL	BETAXOLOL	OXPRENOLOL	METOPROLOL	ATENOLOL	LABETALOL
Cardioselectivity	0	+ +	0	+	+	0
Intrinsic sympathomimetic activity[1]	0	0	+ +	0	0	None α and β blocker
Membrane stabilising effect[2]	+ +	±	+	0	0	0
CNS penetration	+	+	+	0	0	0
Effect on renin release	→	?	→	→	→	→

Notes—1. Sympathomimetic activity in β blocking doses—clinical relevance contested
2. i.e. Local anaesthetic or quinidine-like activity.

ANTI-ARRHYTHMIC DRUGS

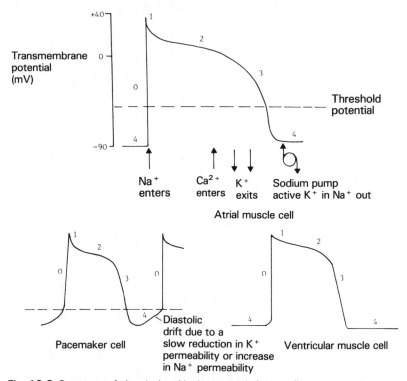

Fig. 13.3 Sequence of electrical and ionic events in heart cells.

Notes
1. Fastest pacemaker drives the heart
2. Vagus (i.e. acetylcholine) slows heart by increasing K^+ permeability and thus decreases diastolic phase 4 drift

Abnormal rhythms result from:

1. *Abnormal automaticity*
   a. Increased firing of pre-existing pacemaker
   b. Emergence of autonomous pacemakers which may occur due to change is slope of phase 4 depolarisation (diastolic drift).

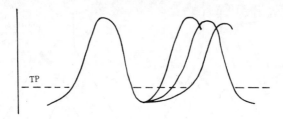

Fig. 13.4 Change in rate of diastolic drift.

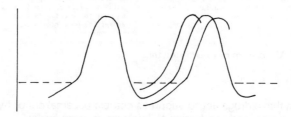

Fig. 13.5 Change in resting membrane potential.

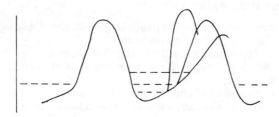

Fig. 13.6 Change in threshold.

2. *Abnormal conduction*
   a. Complete or incomplete block to conduction
   b. Re-entry due to imbalance of conduction velocity and
      refractiveness in branching conduction tissue

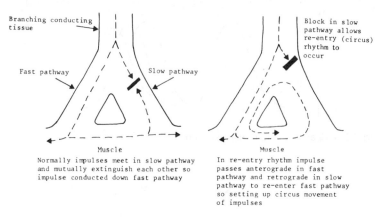

Normally impulses meet in slow pathway
and mutually extinguish each other so
impulse conducted down fast pathway

In re-entry rhythm impulse
passes anterograde in fast
pathway and retrograde in slow
pathway to re-enter fast pathway
so setting up circus movement
of impulses

Fig. 13.7 Mechanism of re-entry rhythm.

Anti-arrhythmic drugs act to suppress ectopic pacemakers or by
speeding or slowing conduction to interrupt re-entry cycles.

MECHANISMS OF ACTION OF ANTI-ARRHYTHMIC DRUGS (VAUGHAN WILLIAMS)

Class I   Inhibit sodium current phase 0, (membrane stabilising) i.e.
lower dV/t of action potential

Class II   Antisympathetic by β-adrenoceptor blockade. No effect on
QRS or QT length. Sinus node and atrial–His conduction are
depressed

Class III   Prolongation of action potential, i.e. prolongation of
effective refractory period and period when fibre is
inexcitable

Class IV   Reduction in inward movement of Ca^{2+} during
depolarisation under circumstances when Na^+ mediated
action potential is suppressed (e.g. ischaemia). This Ca^+
action potential may be responsible for arrhythmias.

Most anti-arrhythmics increase the effective refractory period without
lengthening the duration of the action potential and also depress
phase 4 depolarisation. However class I drugs are divided into three
subgroups:

1A   Slowing of sodium entry with delayed repolarisation and
widening of the action potential

1B   Slowing of sodium entry with accelerated repolarisation and
shortened action potential

1C   Slowing of sodium entry with inhibition of His–Purkinje tissue
and QRS prolongation.

Anti-arrythmic drugs

Class IA	Class II	Class III	Class IV
Quinidine	Propranaolol	Amiodarone	Verapamil
Procaineamide	Atenolol		Diltiazem
Disopyramide	Metoprolol		

Class IB

Lignocaine
Phenytoin
Mexiletine
Tocainide

Class IC

Flecainide
Encainide

CALCIUM ANTAGONISTS

Calcium antagonists block the influx of calcium via slow channels.
Such inflow follows initial depolarisation in heart and smooth muscle.
Because of this basic action, calcium antagonists reduce force of
myocardial contraction, cause coronary and peripheral vascular
dilatation and may reduce contractions in other smooth muscle (e.g.
intestinal).

The members of the group differ in their actions and several
subgroups can be defined on this basis. Two of these are:

Group I   (e.g. diltiazem and verapamil) vasodilators with an
anti-arrhythmic and cardiac depressant effect
Group II   (e.g. nifedipine and nicardipine) predominant vascular
effects.

Clinical uses

Angina: reduce myocardial work and increase coronary blood flow
Hypertension: reduce peripheral vascular resistance
Arrhythmias: verapamil is the drug of choice in terminating
supraventricular tachycardia. It also controls ventricular rate in atrial
fibrillation and flutter
Raynaud's phenomenon: nifedipine may improve the condition.

Toxicity
Flushing, headache, leg oedema, palpitations
Verapamil and diltiazem can cause heart block and asystole
Verapamil can interact with β blockers to produce complete heart
  block, severe hypotension and left ventricular failure
Verapamil causes constipation.

ANTIHYPERTENSIVE DRUGS

1. Commonly used
  a. Diuretics   ⎫ Sodium loss
     (i) Thiazides   ⎬ Vasodilatation
     (ii) Loop diuretics   ⎭ Temporary reduction in blood volume
  b. β blockers   ⎫ Reduce cardiac output
     e.g. metoprolol   ⎪ Inhibit renin release
                             ⎬ ? central action
                             ⎪ ?? inhibit noradrenaline release
                             ⎭ (prejunctional receptor block)
  c. Action on arterioles
     (i) Hydralazine: a vasodilator which causes tachycardia and
         oedema. It is thus given with a β blocker and diuretic.
         Large doses may precipitate a systemic lupus syndrome
     (ii) Calcium antagonists (verapamil, nifedipine, nicardipine,
          amlodipine, isradipine)
  d. Selective α_1 blockers (prazosin, doxazosin, terazosin). May
     cause a rapid fall in blood pressure after the first dose
  e. Angiotension converting enzyme (ACE) inhibitors, (captopril,
     enalapril, fosinopril, lisinopril, perindopril, quinapril, ramipril).
     Inhibit the synthesis of angiotensin II which is a vasoconstrictor
     and which also stimulates aldosterone release (see Ch. 17). It is
     used when diuretics, β blockers and calcium antagonists are
     not tolerated or are not effective. They can cause a rapid fall in
     blood pressure and deterioration in renal function. Blood
     potassium may be raised.

2. More restricted use
  a. Vasodilators: Diazoxide and minoxidil reserved for severe
     resistant hypertension. Sodium nitroprusside is used
     intravenously to control a hypertensive crisis
  b. α_2 agonists reduce noradrenaline release from sympathetic
     nerve endings. Methyldopa can cause sedation and depression
     but can be used during pregnancy and in asthmatics
  c. Non specific α blockers (block α_1, and α_2 receptors) cause
     tachycardia. Phenoxybenzamine is used with a β blocker to
     control hypertension due to a phaeochromocytoma
  d. Sympathetic nerve ending blockers (guanethidine, bethanidine,
     debrisoquine) reserved for severe, resistant hypertension

e. Tyrosine hydroxylase inhibitor (metirosine) inhibits synthesis of catecholamines. It is only used in the management of phaeochromacytoma
f. Ganglion blocker (trimetaphan) is only used to lower the blood pressure during surgery.

ANTI-ANGINAL DRUGS

Drug	Main actions
1. *Nitrates*	Reduction in peripheral resistance
a. Glyceryl trinitrate	Reduction in venous return to heart
b. Isosorbide dinitrate	
2. *β—blockers*	Heart slowing; negative inotropic action
3. *Calcium ion antagonists*	Negative inotropic action; reduction in peripheral resistance; heart slowing (after initial tachycardia) with verapamil and perhexilene, coronary artery dilatation.

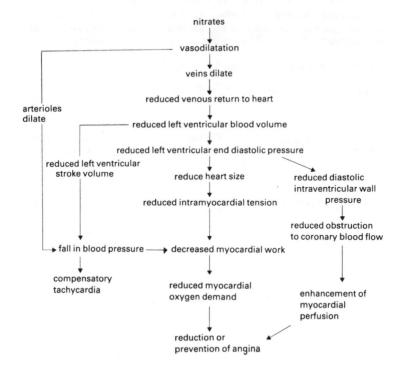

Fig. 13.8 Action of nitrates in angina pectoris.

Mode of action of the nitrites and organic nitrates is via their generation of reactive free radical nitric oxide (NO). This activates guanyl cyclase to form cGMP which in turn stimulates cGMP-dependent protein kinase. The kinase causes dephosphorylation of the light chain of myosin, which is associated with relaxation of smooth muscle and hence arteriolar dilatation.

The antihypertensive drug **hydralazine** probably acts in the same way because it can release nitric oxide.

HEART FAILURE

Drug treatment includes:
1. Diuretics
2. Vasodilators
3. Positive inotropes.

The vasodilators used in heart failure:
Arteriolar dilatation (e.g. nifedipine, hydralazine, ACE inhibitors) reduce afterload by lowering peripheral resistance and left ventricular pressure at systole. This results in improved cardiac output.
Venous dilatation (e.g. nitrates and nitrites) cause opening of capacitance vessels, reduced venous return, reduced left ventricular end-diastolic pressure. This results in less pulmonary congestion.

Rationale of vasodilators use in heart failure

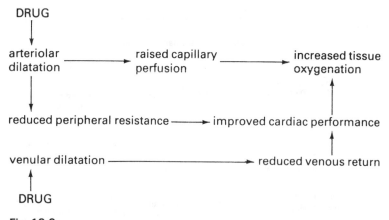

Fig. 13.9

14. Drugs affecting the respiratory system

CENTRAL DEPRESSANTS OF RESPIRATION

Narcotic analgesics
Respiratory depression—reversed by naloxone.

Hypnotics
Profound respiratory depression by most hypnotics including chlormethiazole and alcohol. Relatively less depression by benzodiazepines. Benzodiazepine respiratory depression is reversed by flumazenil. (In hypnotic overdose respiratory failure is treated with assisted ventilation. Central stimulants do more harm than good.)

CENTRAL STIMULANTS OF RESPIRATION

Do not specifically stimulate respiratory centre but are general cerebral stimulants so seizures can occur with excessive dosage.

Doxapram
Ethamivan
} Little used in therapeutics Limited value in respiratory failure complicating acute exacerbations of bronchitis. (Carbon dioxide/oxygen mixture is helpful in treating carbon monoxide poisoning.)

COUGH SUPPRESSANTS

Codeine
Dextromethorphan
Pholcodeine
Isoaminile

Toxicity
1. Respiratory depression
2. Precipitation of respiratory failure in bronchitics and asthmatics
3. Sputum retention

BRONCHOCONSTRICTOR AGENTS

1. Acetylcoline (via M_3 receptors)
2. Histamine
3. Leukotrienes, platelet-activating factor, some prostaglandins (e.g. $PGF_{2\alpha}$)
4. Kinins, substance P
5. Non-adrenergic, non-cholinergic mediators (e.g. purines, excitatory neuropeptides)
6. 5-hydroxytryptamine 5HT
7. β-blockers (in asthmatics).

BRONCHODILATOR AGENTS

1. β agonists (e.g. adrenaline, isoprenaline, salbutamol)
2. Phosphodiesterase inhibitors (e.g. theophylline)
3. Atropine and atropine-like substances (e.g. deptropine)
4. Some prostaglandins—PGE
5. Non-adrenergic, non-cholinergic mediators (e.g. neuroleptics, nitric free radical).

Asthma (potentially reversible airways obstruction)
Asthmatic individuals may show several abnormalities:
1. Circulating IgE (reaginic antibody)
2. Propensity to type I hypersensitivity reactions producing immediate bronchospasm due to allergy. Mast cells degranulate and release histamine, leukotrienes and PAF
3. Immediate bronchospasm in response to stimuli as cold air and sulphur dioxide—possibly due to local nerve reflexes, but mast cell degranulation also involved
4. Prolonged or delayed airways obstruction (late phase reactions) due to an acute inflammatory reaction: oedema of bronchial epithelium, desquamation, infiltration by eosinophils and platelets, plugging with sticky mucus. Due to leukotrienes, PAF, peptide transmitters and possibly local nerve reflexes.

SCHEMES OF DRUG ACTION IN ASTHMA

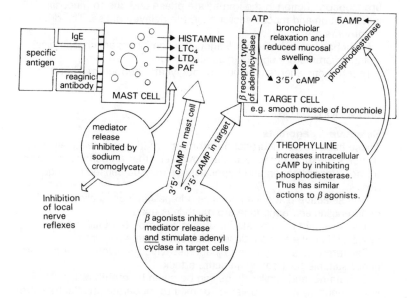

Fig. 14.1 Immediate phase of asthma–drug action.

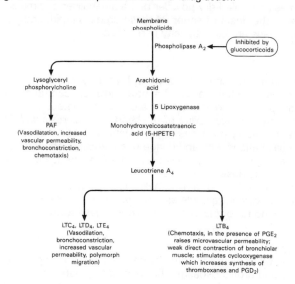

Fig. 14.2 Late phase of asthma–drug action.

The airways obstruction in asthma is mainly due to bronchoconstriction in the immediate phase and due to mucosal inflammation and mucus secretion in the delayed phase. The drug treatments are:
   bronchodilators (selective β agonists; xanthines; anticholinergics)
   anti-inflammatory agents (glucocorticoids)
   prophylactic agents (sodium cromoglycate, nedocromil, ketotifen).

BRONCHODILATORS

Selective β_2 agonists
These have powerful bronchodilator activity (β_2) with relatively little β_1 actions—such as tachycardia. However other β_2 actions including tremor, vasodilatation and hypokalaemia may be caused by large doses.

Non-selective β agonists such as adrenaline, isoprenaline, orciprenaline and ephedrine are much less used.

The selective β_2 agonists include salbutamol, terbutaline and rimiterol. Fenoterol is a little less selective than salbutamol.

Salmeterol is a long acting β_2 agonist which is given twice daily and is not suitable for treating an acute attack.

Salbutamol and similar drugs can be given by mouth or by intravenous injection. However for mild to moderate attacks they are given by pressurised aerosol and inhaled when required. They can also be taken as an inhaled dry powder or via a nebuliser and mask.

When inhaled, the onset of action of these drugs is rapid, and because small doses are used toxicity is reduced.

Xanthines
The main drug in this group is theophylline. It acts by inhibiting phosphodiesterase and thus raising the intracellular concentration of cAMP. Its main pharmacological actions are bronchodilatation, increase in the rate and excitability of the heart, mild diuresis and CNS stimulation. It commonly produces toxic effects such as nausea, insomnia and palpitations. Fits and dangerous cardiac dysrhythmias may result from high doses. There is only a small difference between therapeutic and toxic doses.

Theophylline (in the form of aminophylline) is sometimes given intravenously in severe intractable asthma, but its main use is as a long acting bronchodilator given orally in slow release form.

Anticholinergics
Ipratropium and oxitropium are administered by inhalation in patients with bronchitis and bronchospasm who have not responded adequately to β agonists. They can cause a dry mouth and aggravate glaucoma.

ANTI-INFLAMMATORY AGENTS—act mainly on late phase inflammation

Glucocorticoids (see Fig. 14.2)
These are used in the emergency treatment of severe acute asthma, and on a long-term basis for asthma which has not responded adequately to β_2 agonists.

Oral prednisolone and injected hydrocortisone are used in a severe attack, and in severe chronic asthma long-term oral prednisolone may be needed. However long-term treatment incurs the serious toxic effects of steroids which include adrenal suppression, growth arrest in children, immunosuppression, cataracts and osteoporosis. However, toxicity is greatly reduced if steroids can be given by inhalation. In this way a topical anti-inflammatory action is produced on the respiratory mucosa, but usually little drug is absorbed into the circulation. Also much smaller doses are needed by this route compared with systemic administration. The inhaled steroids may produce oropharyngeal candida infections (due to local immunosuppression) or hoarseness (due to myopathy of the vocal cord muscles). The inhaled glucocorticoids include beclomethasone and budenoside.

PROPHYLACTIC AGENTS

Sodium cromoglycate
Sodium cromoglycate is inhaled and, in some patients, prevents immediate and late phase asthma. It is not used in the treatment of an acute attack. Its mode of action is not completely understood, but it prevents the release of spasmogens from mast cells and reduces local bronchoconstrictor reflexes. Nedocromil has a similar action.

Ketotifen
Ketotifen is an H_1 antihistamine with 5HT blocking activity as well. It aslo inhibits the late phase reaction, possibly by reducing the tissue responsiveness to mediators. Like with other antihistamines, the clinical response to ketotifen is often disappointing.

15. Drugs and the kidney

RENAL TUBULES have four functional zones
Zone I: Proximal tubule
1. Active absorption of 60% of filtered Na^+
2. Accompanying anions to Na^+: 2/3 is Cl^-, 1/3 is HCO_3^-
3. All of filtered K^+ is absorbed
4. Proximal tubular fluid is isosmotic with peritubular fluid.

Zone II: Ascending limb of loop of Henle
1. 25% of filtered Na and Cl are actively absorbed
2. Zone II cells are impermeable to water, thus peritubular fluid is hypertonic.

Zone III: Upper part of ascending limb of loop of Henle (cortical diluting segment) Na^+ continues to be actively absorbed—as in Zone II—but the electrolyte enters the cortical peritubular tissues and not the hypertonic medullary zone. In Zone III the urine becomes progressively more hypotonic.

Zone IV: Distal convoluted tubule and collecting duct
1. Sodium and chloride absorption
2. Secretion of K^+ and H^+ (in exchange for Na^+ absorbed)
3. Water reabsorption (ADH increases water permeability).

DIURETICS (see Tables 15.1 and 15.2)

Drugs which increases the rate of urine production by the kidney:
1. Thiazides
2. High ceiling (loop) diuretics
3. Potassium retaining diuretics:
    a. Spironolactone
    b. Triamterine
    c. Amiloride
4. Osmotic diuretics
Also:
5. Carbonic anhydrase inhibitors—e.g. acetazolamide: not used as a diuretic
6. Xanthines—not used as diuretics (used mainly as bronchodilators). Cause renal vasodilatation and inhibit tubular sodium transport

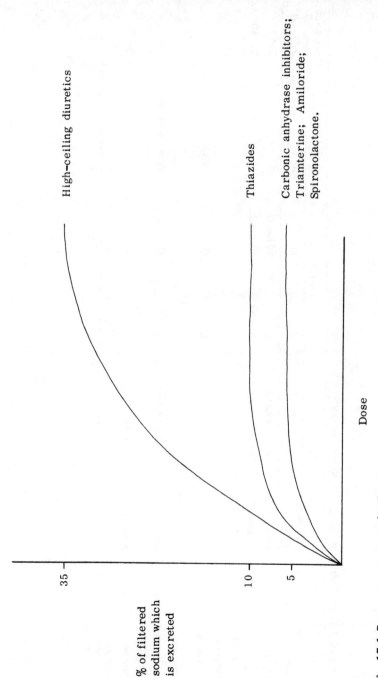

Fig. 15.1 Dose response curves for diuretics.

Table 15.1 Sites of action of diuretics on sodium reabsorption in the nephron

Diuretic	Glomerular filtration	Zone				% Filtered sodium excreted
		I	II	III	IV	
Thiazides	Probably ↓	Minor inhibition	0	Inhibited	0	5–10
Loop (e.g. frusemide)	Possibly ↑	Minor inhibition	Inhibited	Inhibited	0	15–40
Spironolactone Triamterene	0	0	0	0	Inhibited	<5
Amiloride Carbonic anhydrase inhibitors	0	Weak inhibition	0	0	Weak inhibition	<5
Osmotic	Possibly ↑	Inhibited	0	0	0	5–10
Xanthines	↑	0	0	0	0	<5

0 = no effect

Table 15.2 Diuretics

Diuretic	Pharmacokinetics	Toxicity	Uses
THIAZIDES: chlorothiazide hydrochlorothiazide bendrofluazide cyclopenthiazide chlorthalidone (a diuretic sulphonamide—similar properties to thiazides.)	All effective orally Action persists 10 h Action persists 10 h Action persists 20 h Action persists 12 h Action persists 48 h Slowly absorbed	1. Hypokalaemia 2. Hyponatraemia 3. Hypovolaemia (esp. elderly) 4. Hypomagnesaemia 5. Uric acid retention and gout 6. Diminished calcium excretion 7. Reduced glucose tolerance 8. Raised blood lipids 9. Contraction of extracellular volume and secondary polycythaemia.	1. Chronic oedema, especially cardiac 2. Hypertension 3. Diabetes insipidus 4. Idiopathic hypercalciuria.
HIGH CEILING (LOOP) DIURETICS: frusemide ethacrynic acid bumetanide	Rapidly absorbed from gut Also given i.v. Actions persist up to 6 h (bumetanide a little shorter)	1. Hypokalaemia 2. Hyponatraemia 3. Hypovolaemia 4. Hypomagnesaemia 5. Uric acid retention and gout 6. Ototoxicity with high doses 7. Nephrotoxicity with high doses, especially when given with gentamicin or cephaloridine PLUS: (i) For ethacrynic acid: alimentary disturbances and haemorrhage (ii) For bumetanide: muscle pain.	1. Urgent reduction of pulmonary oedema 2. Chronic oedema, especially low output cardiac failure; chronic renal failure 3. Hypercalcaemia 4. Hypertension.

(contd)

Table 15.2 (contd)

Diuretic	Pharmacokinetics	Toxicity	Uses
K⁺ RETAINING DIURETICS: amiloride } non-competitive aldosterone antagonists	Only 20% absorbed from gut Action persists up to 24 h Rapid and complete absorption from gut	1. Potassium retention 2. Uric acid retention.	Diuretic—used with thiazides or loop diuretics to reduce K^+ loss
triamterine }	Action lasts 8–10 h	1. Potassium retention 2. Uric acid retention	Diuretic—used with thiazides or loop diuretics to reduce K^+ loss
spironolactone—competitive aldosterone antagonist	Active metabolite is canrenone which has plasma $t_{1/2} = 10$ h Action lasts 24 h	1. Nausea 2. Potassium retention 3. Weak androgenic actions in women 4. Gynaecomastia in men.	Hypertension. Oedema associated with hyperaldosteronism, especially nephrotic syndrome and hepatic cirrhosis. Not renal failure
OSMOTIC DIURETICS: e.g. mannitol	Given i.v. as a 10 or 20% solution. Brief action	1. Increased plasma volume— precipitation of heart failure 2. Potassium loss.	'Organ dehydration' 1. Closed angle glaucoma 2. Reduction in intracranial pressure—cerebral oedema 3. Forced diuresis.
CARBONIC ANHYDRASE INHIBITORS: e.g. acetazolamide	Well absorbed from gut. Can be given i.v. Action lasts about 8 h	1. Hypersensitivity 2. Blood dyscrasias (uncommon). 3. Renal calculi after prolonged use 4. Potassium loss 5. Mild acidosis.	1. Reduction in formation of aqueous in narrow angle glaucoma 2. Reduction in formation of c.s.f. in benign intracranial hypertension.

Notes:

a. Plasma levels do not give prediction of diuretic effect because of activity of these drugs in kidney tissue (e.g. triamterine plasma $t_{1/2} = 1.5$–2 h, diuresis lasts 8–10 h).

b. A fall in plasma potassium can precipitate coma in patients with liver failure.

7. Demeclocycline—blocks the adenyl cyclase in renal medulla which responds to ADH. Used to treat resistant oedema and during inappropriate secretion of ADH.

Free water clearance and absorption

Free water clearance (C_{H_2O}): that solute-free water that can be removed from the final urine to leave remaining solutes isotonic to plasma.

Free water absorption: amount of water required to make hyperosmotic urine isotonic to plasma, i.e. it is the negative C_{H_2O} which occurs during antidiuresis.

$$C_{H_2O} = V - \frac{\text{urinary osmolality}}{\text{plasma osmolality}} \times V$$

where V is urine flow (ml/min).

CARBONIC ANHYDRASE INHIBITORS

Effects of carbonic anhydrase inhibition
1. Loss of urinary Na^+, K^+, HCO_3^-
2. Systemic acidosis with prolonged use
3. No effect on Cl^- excretion.

Uses of carbonic anhydrase inhibitors
1. Not as diuretics (too weak)
2. Glaucoma (reduces formation of aqueous humour)
3. Intracranial hypertension (reduces c.s.f. formation)
4. Rarely in epilepsy.

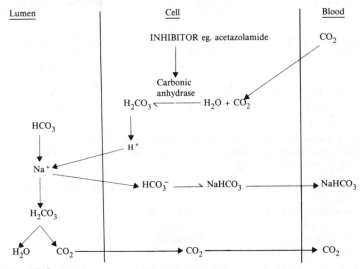

Fig. 15.2

ALTERATION OF URINARY pH

Occasionally necessary in therapeutics.
1. To increase drug elimination in overdose.

Principle

- Non-ionised drug equilibrates rapidly across membranes and can be reabsorbed from renal tubule into blood
- Ionised drug cannot be reabsorbed.

Thus adjusting urinary pH to promote drug ionisation increases urinary drug excretion.
Henderson–Hasselbach equation:

$$pH = pK_a + \log \frac{[A^-]}{[HA]}$$

$[A^-] = H^+$ acceptor; $[HA] = H^+$ donor
so

$$\log \frac{[A^-]}{[HA]} = pH - pK_a$$

NB (a) if pH = pK_a both acids and bases are 50 per cent ionised.
(b) Acids are more ionised when pH > pK_a.
Bases are more ionised when pH < pK_a.

Example   Phenobarbitone pK_a 7.3.

URINE pH 5.3	PLASMA pH 7.3	URINE pH 8.3
$\log \frac{[A^-]}{[HA]} = 5.3 - 7.3$	$\log \frac{[A^-]}{[HA]} = 7.3 - 7.3$	$\log \frac{[A^-]}{[HA]} = 8.3 - 7.3$
$= -2$	$= 0$	$= 1$
$\frac{[A^-]}{[HA]} = 10^{-2}$ $= \frac{0.01}{1}$	$\frac{[A^-]}{[HA]} = 1$ $= \frac{1}{1}$	$\frac{[A^-]}{[HA]} = 10$ $= \frac{10}{1}$

Conclusion The proportion of ionised (and therefore non-reabsorbable) phenobarbitone increases 1000 fold by changing urinary pH from 5.4 to 8.4.

Drugs whose elimination is usefully promoted by manipulation of urinary pH

Alkaline diuresis	Acid diuresis
Barbitone	Amphetamine
Phenobarbitone	Pethidine
Salicylate	

NB Most barbiturates are eliminated by metabolism and are not amenable to forced alkaline diuresis.

2. To increase efficacy of antimicrobials in urine:
   Acid   *Alkali*
   Tetracycline   Streptomycin
   Penicillin   Sulphonamides
3. To discourage growth of certain urinary pathogens, e.g. *E. coli* (alkaline)
4. Symptomatic relief of 'cystitis'
5. To render drugs or metabolites more soluble to prevent crystalluria (e.g. sulphonamides—alkaline) or stone formation (e.g. urate, cystine—alkaline)
6. To replace urinary losses of HCO_3 in renal tubular acidosis.

Drugs for alkalinisation
1. i.v. or oral sodium bicarbonate
2. i.v. sodium lactate (converted to bicarbonate in liver)
3. Oral sodium or potassium citrate.

Drugs for acidification
1. Oral ammonium chloride (converted to ammonia ($\rightarrow$ urea) and HCl)
2. Oral methionine (converted to equivalent of H_2SO_4)
3. Oral arginine hydrochloride (equivalent to HCl)
4. Oral or i.v. ascorbic acid.

Potassium replacement during diuretic therapy
Rarely necessary for uncomplicated hypertension.
Often necessary in heart failure.
1. Good diet, e.g. fruit, meat, providing 80 mmol K^+/day
2. Use of potassium retaining diuretics alone or in combination with other diuretics
3. Potassium supplements as potassium chloride:
   a. Effervescent tablets
   b. Slow release tablets
   May be better retained if not given at same time as diuretic.

Drugs and renal failure
Drugs to avoid or use in reduce dosage in patients with decreased GFR.
1. Drugs excreted unchanged or metabolised by the kidney:
   e.g. allopurinol; penicillins (excreted)
        morphine (metabolised)
   Reduce frequency of administration and dose in proportion to GFR to avoid accumulation and toxicity
2. Nephrotoxins
   e.g. tubular toxins: gentamycin (especially with frusemide); lithium
        interstitial nephritis: NSAID
        crystal formation: tetracyclines, penicillins etc.
   Avoid use in renal impairment

3. ACE inhibitors
   e.g. captopril; enalapril
   Block angiotensin II–dependent
   maintenance of renal perfusion and GFR, especially in renal
      vascular disease
   Avoid in renal artery stenosis
4. Drugs causing K^+ retention
   e.g. oral K^+ supplements
      K^+ sparing diuretics
      sometimes ACE inhibitors (due to inhibition of AII formation)
   Avoid or monitor use. Can cause life-threatening
      hyperkalaemia.

Poisons and haemodialysis

The ability to remove a substance by haemodialysis depends on the
volume of distribution of the substance in the body and the degree of
binding to plasma proteins. Substances that can be removed by
haemodialysis include:
   lithium
   salicylates
   phenobarbitone
   methyl alcohol
   ethyl alcohol
   ethylene glycol.

16. Drugs affecting the gastrointestinal tract

PEPTIC ULCERATION

Two factors determining formation of ulcers:
1. Acid and pepsin secretion
2. Epithelial and mucous resistance.

Drugs can provide:
1. Symptomatic relief only or
2. Promotion of ulcer healing.

H_2 RECEPTOR ANTAGONISTS

These include cimetidine, ranitidine, famotidine and nizatidine.

Actions
Prevent gastrin and vagal stimulation and histamine from enhancing gastric secretion of acid and pepsin. Accelerate healing of peptic ulcer.

Clinical uses
Chronic gastric and duodenal ulceration; peptic oesophagitis; Zollinger–Ellison syndrome.

Toxicity
Diarrhoea, rashes and dizziness. Mild gynaecomastia and impotence (uncommon), confusion in the elderly, inhibition of cytochrome P_{450} oxidative drug metabolism with cimetidine.

Relapse can occur when drug stopped in peptic ulcers: maintenance treatment necessary?

PROTON PUMP INHIBITORS

Omeprazole
Blocks acid secretion from gastric parietal cells by inhibiting H^+K^+-ATPase.

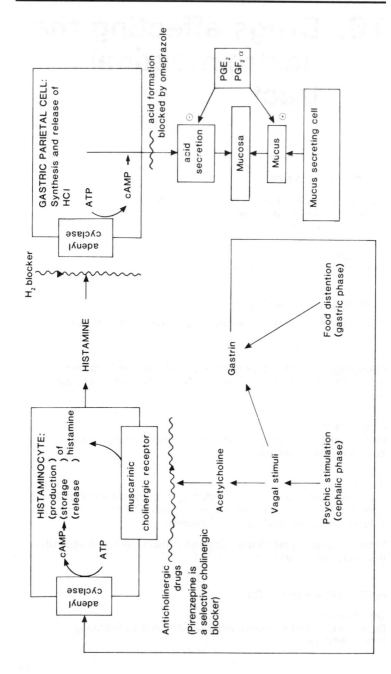

Fig. 16.1 Diagrammatic representation of the relationship between histaminocytes (enterochromaffin-like cells) and parietal cells in the gastric mucosa.

Clinical uses
Benign gastric and duodenal ulceration resistant to H_2 antagonists; Zollinger–Ellison syndrome; reflux oesophagitis.

ANTACIDS

Relief of pain usually without acceleration of healing. If large doses are given (regularly and frequently) may accelerate healing. Act to raise gastric pH and so reduce acid irritation; inactivate pepsin. Two types of antacid:
1. Can cause a systemic alkalosis
    e.g. sodium bicarbonate
2. Without systemic effect
    e.g. calcium carbonate
        aluminium hydroxide
        magnesium carbonate, hydroxide and trisilicate.

Toxicity
Systemic alkalosis and milk–alkali syndrome (hypercalcaemia which in turn may promote acid secretion)
Sodium overload
Aluminium and calcium salts—constipation
Magnesium salts—diarrhoea

ANTICHOLINERGIC DRUGS

Only **pirenzepine** is now used. It promotes healing by inhibition of gastric acid and pepsin secretion through selective aritimuscarinic (M1) effects. Other anticholinergic effects are lacking. The drug may be as effective as H_2 blockers in healing peptic ulcers.

LIQUORICE DERIVATIVES

Carbenoxolone
Increases the rate of healing of gastric ulcers, but less effective with duodenal ulcers. Now seldom used because of side effects related to salt and water retention and hypokalaemia.

PROTECTION OF MUCOSA

Sucralfate
Protects the mucosa against acid attack. The substance is a combination of sulphated sucrose and aluminium hydroxide. It accelerates the healing of gastric and duodenal ulcers.

Tripotassium dicitratobismuthate
Also promotes healing of peptic ulcers. It is a bismuth chelate which physically coats the ulcer crater. Moderately effective against. *Helicobacter pylori*-associated peptic ulceration, especially if combined with antibiotics.

DRUGS WHICH AGGRAVATE PEPTIC ULCERATION
The following may be associated with haemorrhage from ulcers:
1. Aspirin and other NSAI drugs
2. Corticosteroids (unproven as a cause of bleeding)
3. Ethanol
4. Ethacrynic acid
5. Antimitotic drugs.

DRUGS WHICH ENHANCE GASTRIC SECRETION
1. Histamine
2. Betazole—an isomer of histamine with less vascular and cardiac activity
3. Pentagastrin

ANTIEMETIC DRUGS (Table 16.1)

DRUGS WHICH PRODUCE VOMITING
Any drugs (including placebos), but in particular:
1. Cardiac glycosides (e.g. digoxin)
2. Antimitotic agents (e.g. mustine)
3. Dopamine agonists (e.g. levodopa, apomorphine, bromocriptine)
4. Narcotic analgesics (e.g. morphine, diamorphine, pethidine)
5. Gastric irritants (e.g. theophylline, aspirin).

ANORECTIC DRUGS
These drugs are not the answer to obesity.
1. Amphetamine group

	Toxicity
Amphetamine	Dependence, excitation,
Diethylpropion	psychosis, anxiety, tremor,
Phentermine	tachycardia, hypertension.
Mazindol	Tolerance and failure to sustain weight loss.
Fenfluramine	Drowsiness or stimulation, depression, nightmares, tachycardia, hypertension.

2. Bulk agents, e.g. methylcellulose, guar gum. Probably largely ineffective.

Table 16.1 Antiemetic drugs

Drug	Mode of action	Toxicity	Uses
• Anticholinergics: —hyoscine	Antimuscarinic action on the gut and central inhibition of vomiting centre.	Drowsiness, Dry mouth, Blurred vision.	Preoperative medication, Motion sickness.
• Drugs acting on CTZ and gut —Metoclopramide	Increased tone of oesophageal (cardiac) sphincter, increased motility of stomach, reduced transit time of contents through small intestine (due to increased release of acetylcholine). Central inhibition of chemoreceptor trigger zone—on which it acts as a dopamine antagonist.	Extrapyramidal effects including tardive dyskinesias, drowsiness, convulsions in infants following large doses.	Antiemetic, e.g. postoperative, post radiation, drug induced, acceleration of gastric and intestinal emptying. Treatment of spasm and biliary reflux in peptic ulceration.
—Domperidone	Same as metoclopramide.	Less CNS action than metoclopramide.	As for metoclopramide
• Antihistamines (H1): —cyclizine (Marzine) —meclozine (Ancolan) —dimenhydrinate (Dramamine) —promethazine (Phenergan)	Have an anticholinergic hyoscine-like action.	Drowsiness, dry mouth, blurred vision.	Motion sickness and other forms of labyrinthine vomiting.
• Neuroleptics: —Phenothiazines, e.g. chlorpromazine prochlorperazine —Butyrophenones—e.g. haloperidol	Block dopamine receptors in chemoreceptor zone.	Postural hypotension, extrapyramidal effects, ataractic states.	Antiemetic, e.g. postoperative, post radiation, drug induced.
• Betahistine (Serc)	Partial agonist of histamine—exerts vasodilation like histamine, but can relieve histamine headache.	Aggravation of asthma and peptic ulcer. Can produce nausea.	Reduces vertigo and nausea in Menière's disease.
• 5HT$_3$ antagonist Ondansetron	Blocks 5HT$_3$ receptors in gut and CNS.	Constipation, headache.	Reduces nausea and vomiting following anticancer chemotherapy.

APPETITE STIMULATION

1. Any sedative—in particular benzodiazepines and neuroleptics
2. Cyproheptadine: histamine and 5HT receptor blocker
3. Hypoglycaemic agents (insulin and sulphonylureas).

SYMPTOMATIC TREATMENT OF DIARRHOEA

1. Drugs which increase intestinal transit time:
    a. Opiates, e.g. codeine, diphenoxylate
    b. Anticholinergics, e.g. atropine
    c. Loperamide (reduces acetylcholine release)
2. Drugs which increase bulk and viscosity of gut contents, e.g. kaolin, methylcellulose, bran
3. Cholestyramine—effective in diarrhoea due to excess unabsorbed bile salts reaching colon where they cause colonic catharsis. This occurs in:
    a. Diabetic neuropathy affecting gall bladder function
    b. Post-vagotomy (→ increased bile acid secretion)
    c. Ileal resection (→ decreased bile acid reabsorption)
    d. Crohn's disease (→ damage to ileum and decreased bile acid reabsorption)
    Also effective in antibiotic-induced enterocolitis.

PURGATIVES

1. Bulk purgatives

Wheat bran
Contains 30% fibre. This consists of:
1. Cellulose
2. Hemicelluloses
3. Pectins
4. Lignins.

These take up water and so increase the bulk of stools. Stretching the colonic wall stimulates peristalis, thus reducing transit time. Wheat fibre binds to bile salts and increases their excretion. However, the blood cholesterol is not reduced on a bran-supplemented diet, although this does occur on ingesting guar gum or fruit pectin.
   Bran is of value in treating:
1. Constipation
2. Diverticulosis
3. Spastic colon.
Other applications that have been suggested (e.g. haemorrhoids, anal fissures, diverticular disease, preventing carcinoma of the colon, obesity, coronary artery disease) are speculative.
Other bulk agents—Methylcellulose; frangula bark; guar gum; pectins.

2. Osmotic agents
3. Chemical stimulants ('irritants') } see Table 16.2
4. Lubricants and stool softeners.

Toxicity
1. Flatulence
2. Reduced absorption of calcium.

DRUG-INDUCED JAUNDICE AND LIVER DAMAGE

The principal mechanisms of drug-induced jaundice may be grouped as follows:
1. Haemolysis
2. Competition for binding of bilirubin to plasma proteins (e.g. sulphonamides, salicylates)
3. Competition for binding of bilirubin to cell proteins (e.g. flavaspidic acid—the active principle of male fern extract anthelmintics)
4. Competition for glucuronide-forming enzymes (e.g. novobiocin)
5. Intrahepatic cholestasis due to competition for biliary canalicular excretory mechanisms (e.g. rifampicin)
6. Intrahepatic cholestasis due to alterations in the canalicular membrane (e.g. C17 alkyl testosterone derivatives, such as methyltestosterone and norethandrolone, oestrogens and progestogens of the pill)
7. Diffuse hepatic damage (e.g. carbon tetrachloride).

Hypersensitivity may account for many instances of drug-induced jaundice. It can be associated with other features such as rashes, fever arthralgia and eosinophilia. The reaction is not dose-related, affects only a small number of patients taking the drug and is commoner after multiple exposures.

The drugs most commonly reported as being associated with jaundice are:
1. Halothane — Hepatitis
2. Phenelzine, iproniazid, isocarboxazid — Hepatitis
3. α-methyldopa — Hepatitis. Rarely haemolysis
4. Chlorpromazine and other phenothiazines — Stasis with hepatitis
5. Imipramine, amitriptyline, iprindole — Stasis with hepatitis
6. Benzodiazepines — Stasis with hepatitis
7. Phenylbutazone, oxyphenbutazone, indomethacin — Stasis with hepatitis
8. Isoniazid — Hepatitis
9. PAS, rifampicin, ethambutol, pyrazinamide — Stasis with hepatitis

Table 16.2 Other purgatives

Drug	Pharmacological properties	Approximate dose effect interval	Toxicity*	Special uses
Osmotic purgatives	Largely unabsorbed from gut and so osmotically active.			
SODIUM SULPHATE	Increased bulk of water in lumen stimulates peristalsis.	2 h		
MAGNESIUM SULPHATE	Acts like sodium sulphate, but in addition magnesium ion stimulates peristalsis by liberating cholecystokinin.	2 h	Magnesium can be absorbed and be of clinical significance in renal failure	Hepatocellular failure.
LACTULOSE (Duphalac)	Is a disaccharide which is split by bacteria in colon to organic acids which are unabsorbed and act osmotically to increase bulk of stools. Gas formation is increased.	48 h	Contraindicated in galactosaemia	Hepatocellular failure.
Chemical stimulants of colonic action ('irritants')				
CASTOR OIL	Digested in small intestine to ricinoleic acid. Can stimulate uterine contractions at full term.	2 h	Excessive loss of water and electrolytes (including potassium).	Obsolete
SENNA	Contains glycosides which are hydrolysed by colonic bacteria to sennosides A and B. These are absorbed and then stimulate colonic peristalsis by acting on mural nerve plexuses. Enters milk.	8 h	Griping and diarrhoea. Diarrhoea in suckling child. Melanosis coli. Red or yellow colouration of urine.	

Drug				
BISACODYL	Deacetylated in gut, absorbed, glucuronidated in liver and enters enterohepatic circulation. Has a direct action on gut wall to stimulate peristalsis. Also absorbed into circulation and reaches gut wall in arterial blood.	10 h		Can be given by suppository.
PHENOLPHTHALEIN	15% absorbed from gut, excreted in bile and undergoes an enterophepatic circulation—resulting in a prolonged effect. Active fraction produced in liver and undergoes further modification in colon.	8–10 h	4% develop a fixed drug eruption. Other rashes. SLE-like syndrome. Alkaline urine coloured pink.	Obsolete
Lubricants and stool softeners:				
DIOCTYL SODIUM SULPHOSUCCINATE (DSS; DIOCTYL)	Surface acting agent which allows water to enter inspissated colonic contents.	1 d	Detegent action alters intestinal mucosa permeability.	Faecal impaction
LIQUID PARAFFIN	Lubricates contents of colon. Not digested.	1 d	Interferes with absorption of fat soluble vitamins. Aspiration lipid pneumonia. Anal leakage. Absorption into tissues (e.g. after intestinal operations). Can cause granuloma formation. Possible carcinogenicity.	Obsolete

*All can give rise to purgative abuse syndrome: dilated, atonic colon; sodium depletion; potassium depletion; enteropathy and weight loss; osteomalacia.

10. Tetracycline   Direct hepatocellular
                                              toxicity: fatty liver
11. Erthromycin, ampicillin,
    sulphonamides, nitrofurantion   Stasis with hepatitis
12. Chlorpropamide, tolbutamide   Stasis with hepatitis
13. Combined contraceptive pill   Pure cholestasis
14. Methotrexate   Cirrhosis
15. Oxyphenisatin   Chronic active hepatitis.

17. Pharmacology of the endocrine system

Soluble protein and peptide hormones
Soluble in body fluids in free form

Short $t_{1/2}$, e.g. TSH, ACTH, (10–20 min); insulin and catecholamines (1–2 min), therefore plasma levels fluctuate rapidly

Usually act via effect on membrane bound adenyl cyclase and alteration of cyclic AMP

Examples Parathormone
Calcitonin
GH, FSH, ACTH, TSH, ADH
Insulin, glucagon
Catecholamines
Angiotensin II

Hydrophobic small molecule hormones
Carried by albumin or specific transport proteins in plasma, e.g. transcortin

Longer $t_{1/2}$, e.g. cortisol (1 h); thyroxine (1 week) therefore plasma levels relatively constant

Usually act by binding to cytoplasmic or nuclear receptor molecules

Examples: Cortisol
Thyroxine
Testosterone
Oestrogens
Progesterone

HYPOTHALAMUS

Table 17.1 Drugs influencing releasing factors (see Table 17.2)

	GRF	CRF	LHRH	PIF
Acetylcholine		+	+	
Noradrenaline	+	+	+	
Dopamine	+		+	
5-HT	+	+		
Phenothiazines				–
Prostaglandin E$_2$				+
Ergotamine				+

+ = stimulates release of releasing factors
– = inhibits release of releasing factors

151

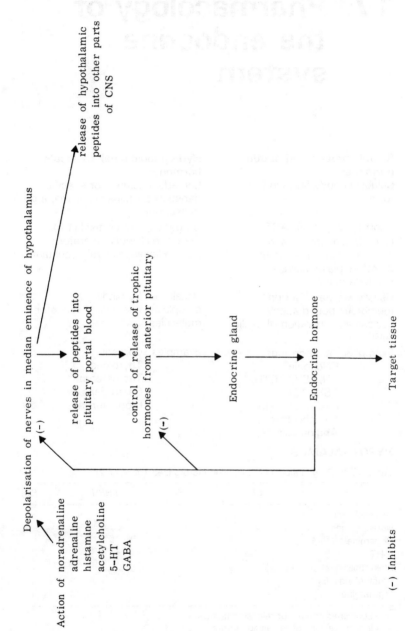

(–) Inhibits

Fig. 17.1

Table 17.2 Hypothalamic releasing and inhibiting factors

	Hypothalamic peptide	Action on anterior pituitary
Peptides isolated	Thyrotrophin releasing hormone (TRH).	Thyrotrophin (TSH) released. Prolactin released.
	Luteinising hormone releasing hormone (LHRH).	Luteinising hormone (LH) released Follicle stimulating hormone (FSH) released.
	Somatostatin (SRIF; GHRIH).	Inhibits release of growth hormone (GH). Inhibits release of TSH. Also inhibits insulin, glucagon and gastrin secretion.
	Dopamine (prolactin inhibitory hormone).	Inhibits release of prolactin.
	Corticotrophin releasing factor (CRF).	ACTH released.
	GH releasing factor (GHRF).	GH released.
Peptide thought to exist	Prolactin releasing factor (apart from TRH) (PRF).	Prolactin released.

The release of prolactin from the pituitary is usually physiologically inhibited by prolactin inhibiting factor (PIF) which is dopamine.

ANTERIOR PITUITARY HORMONES

Peptide hormone	MW
Growth hormone (GH)	21 000
Prolactin	Similar structure to GH
Gonadotrophins (LH and FSH)	Each 30 000
Corticotrophin (ACTH)	45 000

POSTERIOR PITUITARY HORMONES

(Both contain amino acids)

Vasopressin	1083
Oxytocin	1007

ANTERIOR PITUITARY

GROWTH HORMONE

Excess GH → gigantism; acromegaly. Deficiency → dwarfism.

Increase in secretion caused by:
1. Slow wave sleep
2. Fasting, hypoglycaemia, stress
3. L-dopa
4. Amphetamine
5. GHRF.

Decrease in secretion caused by:
1. Glucose, protein consumption
2. Corticosteroids
3. Somatostatin.

Actions
1. Promotes protein synthesis
2. Synergistic effect with insulin, in increasing amino acid flow into cells
3. Stimulates somatomedin secretion by the liver which mediates skeletal growth.

Use
Growth failure in children due to GH lack.

Block of excessive GH production
Bromocriptine
Somatostatin analogues.

PROLACTIN

Hyperprolactinaemia → impotence, hypogonadism and
gynaecomastia in men.
→ amenorrhoea, anovulation, galactorrhoea
in women.

Increase in secretion caused by:
1. Stress
2. Sleep
3. Orgasm
4. Neuroleptics ⎱ act by antagonising
5. Reserpine   ⎰ dopamine effects
6. Metoclopramide
7. TRH and PRF.

Decrease in secretion caused by:
1. Dopamine
2. Bromocriptine, L-dopa, pergolide, metergoline, apomorphine.

Actions
1. Mammotropic
2. Lactogenic
3. In large amounts affects sex function.

Bromocriptine
Dopamine receptor agonist which reduces prolactin secretion.

Uses
1. Inhibition of purperal lactation
2. Hyperprolactinaemia in male and female hypogonadism
3. Galactorrhoea
4. Acromegaly
5. Parkinsonism.

Toxicity
1. Nausea, vomiting, syncope
2. Constipation
3. Cramps
4. Dystonia
5. Hallucinations.

GONADOTROPHINS

Actions

FSH	LH
In female:	
development primary ovarian follicle; granulosa cell proliferation; increases oestrogen production	induces ovulation; stimulates thecal oestrogen production; initiates and maintains corpus luteum
In male:	
increases spermatogenesis	stimulates androgen production by Leydig cells

Gonadotrophins in therapy
FSH and LH in human menopausal urinary gonadotrophin (HMG)
LH in human chorionic gonadotrophin (HCG)
FSH pure preparation.

Uses
1. Primary and secondary amenorrhoea
2. Polycystic ovary syndrome
3. Stimulation of spermatogenesis in secondary testicular failure
4. Undescended testis.

Stimulation of gonadotrophin secretion by clomiphene

Uses
1. To treat infertility in female
2. Polycystic ovary syndrome
3. Undescended testes.

Inhibition of gonadotrophin secretion by danazol or LHRH analogues

Uses
1. Gynaecomastia in males
2. Precocious puberty in females
3. Endometriosis
4. Fibrocystic mastitis.

ACTH (CORTICOTROPHIN)

Peptide of 39 amino acids.

Tetracosactrin (synthetic) contains the first 24 of these and has same activity.
The remaining 15 are species specific and related to antigenic activity.
    Deficiency contributes to Simmond's disease.
    Excess produces Cushing's disease.

Actions
1. Increase size and metabolic activity of adrenal cortex
2. Mainly stimulation of synthesis and release of cortisol from adrenal
3. Also increases synthesis and release of:
    a. Other corticosteroids
    b. Sex hormones
    c. Aldosterone (minor effect).

Uses and toxicity
Mainly as for cortisol, except that corticotrophin does not produce adrenal suppression and does not arrest linear growth in children but may stimulate androgen production.

POSTERIOR PITUITARY

VASOPRESSIN (ANTIDIURETIC HORMONE; ADH)

Released by:
1. Increased plasma osmotic pressure
2. Decreased blood volume
3. Emotional stress
4. Morphine, nicotine
5. Carbamazepine.

Actions
1. Increase in water reabsorption by the distal tubules and collecting ducts of the kidney
2. Vasoconstriction
3. Contraction of smooth muscle—increase in intestinal peristalsis
4. Lowering of pressure in the portal vein.

Uses
Given by injection (absorbed from nasal mucosa, but snuff can cause rhinitis, bronchospasm and pulmonary fibrosis) for:
1. Bleeding oesophageal varices
2. Cranial diabetes insipidus.

Toxicity of injected vasopressin
1. Pallor, colic, bowel evacuation
2. Increase in blood pressure, angina
3. Reduced hepatic blood flow.

Synthetic lysine vasopressin (LVP) Nasal spray effective in diabetes insipidus. No nasal or pulmonary irritation (c.f. ADH).
1-desamino-8-D arginine vasopressin (DDAVP) Synthetic long-acting analogue of ADH. Drug of choice in diabetes insipidus because no vasoconstriction, smooth muscle contraction or respiratory irritation. Also has a role in variceal and uraemic bleeding. Given nasally or by injection.

The *thiazide diuretics* are used in nephrogenic diabetes insipidus. They act by reducing glomerular blood flow.

OXYTOCIN

Released by
1. Suckling
2. Emotional stimuli.

Actions
1. Contraction of fundus of uterus
2. Contraction of mammary gland ducts.

Uses
(Usually given parenterally, but absorbed via nasal or buccal mucosae)
1. Initiation of labour
2. Control of post-partum haemorrhage.

Toxicity
1. Excessive uterine contractions and rupture of uterus
2. Water retention
3. Neonatal jaundice
4. Hypotension.

Synthetic oxytocin—pure and not contaminated with vasopressin.

SEX HORMONES

TESTIS

Main androgen is testosterone produced by Leydig cells. This enters target cells and is converted in the nuclei to the more active androgen dihydrotestosterone. Both testosterone and dihydrotestosterone are inactivated in the liver.

Main actions of androgens
1. Development of male secondary sex characteristics
2. Nitrogen retention, growth and bone maturation, muscle development
3. Temporal recession of hair line
4. Sebum secretion
5. Spermatogenesis and seminal fluid formation.

LH stimulates testosterone secretion by Leydig cells
FSH stimulates spermatogenesis in seminiferous tubules

Androgenic substances (used in replacement therapy)
1. Testosterone esters
2. Fluoxymesterone
3. Mesterolone.

Less virilising androgens (used as anabolic substances in renal failure, osteoporosis etc.)
1. Nandrolone
2. Methandienone.

Cyproterone
An anti-androgen with progestogenic activity. Competes with testosterone for target organ receptors. Blocks synthesis of testosterone (and oestrogens). Blocks gonadotrophin release.

Uses
1. Unacceptable sexual activity in males
2. Precocious puberty
3. Acne and hirsutism in females.

OVARY

Main hormones
1. Oestradiol ⎱ secreted by theca interna and
2. Oestrone ⎰ stratum granulosum
3. Progesterone—secreted by corpus luteum (with a small amount of androgens).

Oestrogen actions
1. Development of female secondary sex characteristics
2. Female distribution of fat, weak anabolic activity
3. Proliferation of endometrium
4. Ductal growth of breast with stromal and acinar development.

Progesterone actions
1. Secretory activity in endometrium
2. Viscid secretion by endocervical glands
3. Contributes to acinar development of breast.

Receptors for oestrogens and progestogens occur in cytoplasm and hormone—receptor complex travels to nucleus to influence cell metabolism, growth and division.
Oestrogen pretreatment increases mass of progesterone receptor.

Gonadotrophins
1. FSH stimulates maturation of ovarian follicles and release of oestrogen
2. LH stimulates progesterone release
3. Plasma oestrogen inhibits FSH and LH release ⎱ by inhibiting gonadotrophin
4. Plasma progesterone inhibits LH release. ⎰ releasing hormone production in the hypothalamus

OESTROGENS

Ethinyl oestradiol	Synthetic. Well absorbed orally. $t_{1/2}$ = 24 h
Diethyl stilboestrol	Synthetic. Well absorbed orally As active as oestradiol but longer acting
Oestradiol-17β	The most potent natural oestrogen. Largely oxidised to oestrone and then hydrated to form oestriol These three active substances are excreted as conjugates.

Uses
1. Contraception
2. Replacement therapy
3. Functional uterine haemorrhage
4. Neoplastic disease, e.g. prostatic carcinoma.

Oestrogen antagonist—tamoxifen, is used for treatment of breast cancer.

PROGESTOGENS

Progesterone	Considerable first pass metabolism, therefore usually injected or given sublingually. Excreted as pregnanediol and pregnanolone
Norethisterone	Synthetic progestogen. Rapidly absorbed orally. $t_{1/2} = 8$ h
Norethindrone	Some androgenic action and should not be used in threatened abortion
Dydrogesterone	Not oestrogenic or androgenic. Does not suppress ovulation

Uses
1. Contraception
2. Functional uterine haemorrhage and other menstrual abnormalities
3. Dysmenorrhoea
4. Endometriosis
5. Threatened abortion
6. Delaying menstruation (e.g. for weddings, sporting events).

THE ORAL CONTRACEPTIVE 'PILL'

The combined pill consists of an oestrogen plus a progestogen.

Action of oestrogen
1. Suppresses ovulation by inhibition of gonadotrophin release due to suppression of hypothalamic releasing factor
2. Oestrogens may also affect transport of ovum along fallopian tube.

Actions of progestogen
1. Pseudodecidual change in endometrium prevents implantation of zygote
2. Modification of cervical mucus makes it impenetrable to sperm.

Endocrine and metabolic effects of combination
1. Absence of premenstrual rise and midcycle peaks of LH and FSH
2. Absence of late cycle rise of progesterone
3. Increase in thyroid binding globulin and protein bound iodine
4. Reduced carbohydrate tolerance
5. Increased triglycerides, total cholesterol and reduced high density lipoprotein.

Side effects associated with different types of steroid in contraceptive pill

Oestrogen	Progestogen	Both
Breakthrough bleeding	Acne	Hypertension
Carbohydrate intolerance	Depression	Irregular bleeding
Cerebral arterial	Hirsutism	Myocardial infarction
thrombosis	Reduced libido	Post-pill
Cervical erosion	Vaginal dryness	amenorrhoea
Cloasma		
Cholestatic jaundice		
Depression		
Menstrual cramps		
Migraine		
Oedema		
Vaginal discharge		
Vaginal candidiasis		
Venous thrombosis		

Low dose progesterone-only preparations
Reduced effectiveness because ovulation is not constantly suppressed and main action is on cervical mucus.
No serious adverse effects, but often produces:
1. Irregular uterine bleeding
2. Breast tenderness
3. Skin flushing
4. Headaches.

Deaths attributable to contraceptive method
—plus those due to pregnancies (per 100 woman years)
—higher in smokers and those with familial cardiovascular problems

Age	20–34 years	35–44 years
'Pill'	0.002–0.004	0.02
IUD	0.002–0.004	0.002
Occlusive devices	0.002–0.004	0.002

THYROID GLAND

Thyroid secretes 3 hormones:
1. Thyroxin (T_4)
2. Triiodothyronine (T_3)
3. Calcitonin.

THYROID HORMONE BIOSYNTHESIS

Excessive production of T_3 and T_4 produces thyrotoxicosis; deficiency produces myxoedema or cretinism.

Table 17.3 Risk related to method of contraception

Method of contraception	Excess of admissions to hospital (per 100 woman years)		Pregnancies (per 100 woman years)	Fate of pregnancies			
				Full term	Spontaneous abortion	Ectopic	Terminations
Combined oestrogen-progestogen pill	Stroke	0.035	0.36	0.2	0.045	0.01	0.094
	Venous thrombosis and embolus	0.07					
	Myocardial infarction	0.01					
IUD	Uterine perforations	0.05	2.0	0.495	0.755	0.12	0.605
	Pelvic inflammatory disease	0.2					
Occlusive devices	Nil		5.0	3.045	0.64	0.02	1.295

Other considerations:
1. 'Pill'. Increased risk of hypertension, cervical erosion and carcinoma, and possibly of uterine carcinoma and hepatocellular adenoma. Effect on breast cancer unknown. Suppression of menstrual disorders, fewer benign breast lesions, fewer ovarian cysts
2. IUD. Migration of the device into the peritoneum; intestinal obstruction with copper devices
3. Occlusive methods. Reduced chance of pre-invasive carcinoma of cervix and venereal disease.

Secretion of T_3 and T_4 increased by: TSH (released in response to low plasma levels of T_3 and T_4); immunoglobulins with TSH activity.

Actions of T_3 and T_4

Hormone action	Clinical consequence
1. Stimulation of metabolism	Heat intolerance, increased appetite with weight loss, raised metabolic rate in hyperthyroidism; coma and hypothermia in hypothyroidism
2. Promotion of growth and development	Dwarfism and mental deficiency in cretinism (neonatal hypothyroidism)

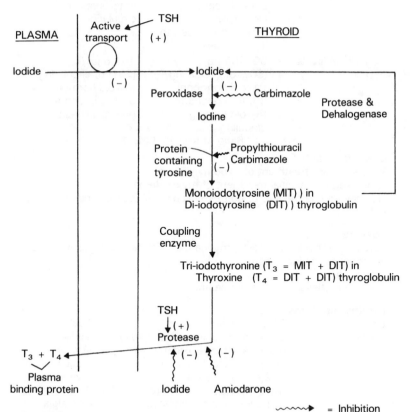

Fig. 17.2

Hormone action	Clinical consequence
3. Sensitisation to sympathetic effects and to catecholamines due to development of extra β receptors.	Eyelid retraction, tachycardia, atrial fibrillation, tremor, hyperactive reflexes in hyperthyroidism; delayed relaxation of reflexes in hypothyroidism.

Pharmacokinetics

	T_4	T_3
Gut absorption	Complete	Complete
Latency before action starts	24 h	6 h
Peak effect	7–10d	24 h
$t_{1/2}$	6–7d	2d or less
Metabolism	Conjugation and enterohepatic circulation 20% is converted to T_3 in tissues	Conjugation and enterohepatic circulation
Normal levels	50–100 µg/l (80% of circulating thyroid hormone) 99.95% bound to thyroid binding globulin	1–1.6 µg/l (20% of circulating thyroid hormone) 99.5% bound to plasma protein

Ratio of free T_4:T_3 is 4–5:1

Uses of T_3 and T_4
T_4 is standard treatment of hypothyroidism.
T_3 is used in the initial treatment of myxoedema coma.
(T_4 may reduce the size of goitres which have not responded to iodine alone.)

Toxicity
Cardiac—tachycardia, angina, myocardial infarction, congestive failure, arrhythmias, sudden death.
Diarrhoea.
Tremor, restlessness, heat intolerance.

Antithyroid drugs

Drug	Mode of action	Toxicity
Carbimazole	Blockade of iodination of tyrosyl residues; inhibits oxidation of iodine in thyroid gland. Delay of 1–2 months before hyperthyroidism begins to respond. Active metabolite is methimazole	Rashes Marrow depression— very rare Drug fever Arthralgia

Propylthiouracil	Blockade of iodination of tyrosyl residues in thyroid gland. Delay of 1–2 months before hyperthyroidism responds	Rashes Marrow depression— very rare
^{131}I and ^{125}I	Concentrated in thyroid gland by thyroid trap. Isotopes irradiate and destroy thyroid cells	Under or over treatment

Actions of iodine

Essential part of T_3 and T_4 molecules.
Prevents simple non-toxic goitre.
In thyrotoxicosis:
1. Reduces vascularity of thyroid
2. Reduces release of T_3 and T_4. } for 1–2 weeks only

β—adrenergic blockers

Therapeutically useful to control tremor and tachycardia in thyrotoxicosis.

PARATHYROID HORMONE AND CALCIUM

Plasma calcium controlled by:
1. Parathyroid hormone (PTH)
2. Active vitamin D hormone (1.25–DHCC). } both raise plasma Ca^{++}
Calcitonin lowers plasma calcium, but the physiological importance of this is not understood.

Dihydrotachysterol (AT10)
A synthetic substance which is related to vitamin D and raises plasma Ca^{++} in a similar way.

1-α-hydroxycholecalciferol (alphacalcidol)
Synthetic preparation equivalent to 1,25-DHCC, for use in patients with failure to convert inactive to active form of vitamin D due to renal disease.

MAIN ACTIONS OF PTH, 1,25-DHCC AND CALCITONIN

Hormone	*Actions*	*Mode of Action*
PTH (released when plasma Ca^{++} falls or PO_4^- rises)	*Kidney:* (i) Phosphaturia and increased tubular reabsorption of Ca^{++}. (ii) Increased conversion of 25-HCC to 1,25-DHCC. *Bone*: Increased Ca^{++} mobilisation.	(i) Activation of adenyl cyclase, increase in renal tubular cAMP. (ii) Activation of renal 1-α-hydroxylase. Activation of adenyl cyclase, increase in bone cAMP. Increased osteoblast activity.

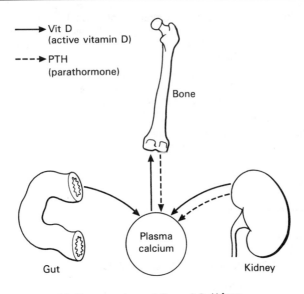

Vit D : promotes net flow of Ca^{++} from
gut + kidney → bone

PTH : promotes net flow of Ca^{++} from
bone + kidney → blood

Fig. 17.3 Regulation of calcium metabolism by vitamin D and parathyroid hormone.

Hormone	Actions	Mode of Action
1,25-DHCC	*Gut:* Increased Ca^{++} absorption. *Bone:* Increases turnover—Ca^{++} mobilised and is used for mineralisation of new bone. *Kidney:* Minor role in increasing tubular reabsorption of Ca^{++}.	Formation of calcium binding protein. Stimulation of active transport of Ca^{++} across osteocyte plasma membrane.
CALCITONIN	*Bone:* Antagonises actions of PTH. *Kidney:* Promotes excretion of PO$_4$, Ca, Na.	Slows osteoclastic bone absorption and increases calcium deposition by osteoblasts.

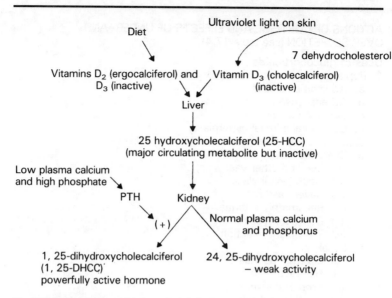

Fig. 17.4 Metabolic activation of vitamin D.

ADRENAL CORTEX

SECRETIONS

1. Glucocorticoids: mainly cortisol + some corticosterone
2. Mineralocorticoids: mainly aldosterone and some deoxycorticosterone
3. Small amounts of sex hormones: testosterone, androsterone, oestrogens, progesterone.

SECRETION OF CORTISOL AND ITS PHARMACOKINETICS

1. Cortisol synthesis and release under ACTH control
2. Diurnal variation of cortisol levels reflects ACTH release—peak level at about 8:00 and trough at midnight
3. Feedback inhibition of ACTH release and CRF secretion by circulating cortisol
4. 95% of cortisol bound in circulation to corticosteroid binding globulin (CBG; transcortin)
5. The level of CBG also varies: maximum binding at midnight and minimum at about 8:00
   a. $t_{1/2}$ of cortisol in plasma = 2h
   b. $t_{1/2}$ of actions of cortisol = 8–12h
6. Well absorbed from gut (but *cortisone* shows variable absorption and some patients with liver disease may fail to activate it to cortisol).

ACTIONS OF CORTISOL AND EFFECTS OF UNDER- AND
OVER-SECRETION (see table 17.4)

Uses of glucocorticoids
1. Replacement
    a. Addison's disease
    b. Adrenal crisis
    c. Simmond's disease
    d. Congenital adrenal hyperplasia
2. Suppression of inflammatory and immune disease
    a. Systemic
        (i)   SLE and other vasculitis,
        (ii) Acute anaphylaxis
        (iii) Severe asthma
        (iv) Rheumatoid arthritis
        (v)   Dermatomyositis
        (vi) Transplant rejection
    b. Local
        (i)   Eczema, psoriasis
        (ii) Hay fever
        (iii) Bronchial asthma
        (iv) Local joint disease
        (v)   Iritis
3. Feedback inhibition of pituitary
    Congenital adrenal hyperplasia.

See also Table 17.5

ALDOSTERONE
Main mineralocorticoid of adrenal cortex.

Excessive secretion (as in Conn's syndrome)
Sodium retention (and hypertension), potassium loss (and muscular
weakness). May have oedema but not a constant feature.

Diminished secretion
Part of the picture of Addison's disease (contributes to
hyponatraemia, hyperkalaemia, hypovolaemia and hypotension).

Control of secretion
Transient stimulation by ACTH (but in pituitary failure aldosterone
secretion continues).
Main stimulation to secretion:
1. Low plasma Na^+
2. Raised plasma K^+
3. Raised plasma angiotensin II.

Table 17.4 Actions of cortisol and consequences of under and over secretion

	Actions	Deficiency	Excess
Carbohydrate, protein and fat metabolism	Raises blood sugar by enhanced gluconeogenesis and insulin antagonism; redistributes body fat centrally and raises blood cholesterol; decreases protein synthesis e.g. in muscles and skin	Hypoglycaemia Loss of weight	Cushing's syndrome. Weight gain; increase in trunk fat; moon face; skin striae, bruising, atrophy; wasting of limb muscles; delayed healing.
Water and salt metabolism	Inhibits fluid shift from extracellular to intracellular compartment; antagonises vasopressin action on kidney; increases vasopressin destruction and decreases its production. Sodium and water retention, potassium loss.	Loss of weight Hypovolaemia Hyponatraemia	Oedema, thirst, polyuria. Hypertension. Muscular weakness.
Haematological	Lowers lymphocyte and eosinophil counts and raises polymorph count; increases RBC, platelets and clotting tendency.		Florid complexion and polycythaemia.
Alimentary	Increased production of gastric acid and pepsin.	Anorexia and nausea	Dyspepsia; aggravation of peptic ulcer.
CVS	Sensitises arterioles to catecholamines, enhances production of angiotensinogen. Fall in high density lipoprotein with increased total cholesterol.	Hypotension, fainting	Hypertension. Atherosclerosis.
Skeletal	Decreased production of cartilage and bone; anti-vitamin D; increased renal loss of calcium.		Backache due to osteoporosis. Dwarfing in children (also anti-G.H. effect).
Nervous system	Altered neuronal excitability. Inhibition of uptake of catecholamines.		Depression and other mood changes.
Anti-inflammatory	Reduces formation of fluid and cellular exudate; reduces fibrous tissue repair.		
Immunological	Large doses lyse lymphocytes and plasma cells (transient release of immunoglobulin).		Reduced lymphocyte mass. Diminished immunoglobulin production. Immune suppression and lowered resistance to infections
Feedback	Inhibits release of ACTH and MSH.	Pigmentation of skin and mucosa	

Table 17.5 Relative activities of glucocorticoids and mineralocorticoids

	Compared with cortisol (w/w)		Special features
	Mineralocorticoid activity	Glucocorticoid and anti-inflammatory activity	
Prednisolone	× 0.8	× 4	$t_{1/2}$ = 2.5–3h. Mainly used for anti-inflammatory actions.
6-α-methyl prednisolone	× 0.5	× 5	
Triamcinolone (9-α-fluoro-16-α-hydroxy prednisolone)	0	× 5	Can produce flushes, sweating and muscular weakness. Arthritis on withdrawal. Plus glucocorticoid side effects. Used as an anti-inflammatory.
Betamethasone (9-α-fluoro-16-α-methyl prednisolone)	0	× 25	Used for anti-inflammatory actions.
Dexamethasone (9-α-fluoro-16-α-methyl prednisolone)	0	× 25	Used for anti-inflammatory actions.
Fludrocortisone	× 125	× 10	Used for its mineralocorticoid activity in hypoadrenal states.
Aldosterone	× 1000	0	Has to be injected. Not often used clinically.

Actions

Reduced loss of Na^+
Enhanced loss of K^+ and H^+ at:
1. Zone IV in distal renal tubule
2. Sweat glands
3. Gut wall.

RENIN

A number of different proteins (MW 40 000) which split angiotensin I from circulating renin substrate.

Located in granules in epithelioid or juxtaglomerular (JG) cells of renal afferent artery.

Hypotheses of renin release (not mutually exclusive):
1. Regulation by sympathetic nerves via β-adrenergic receptors (so release blocked by β-blockers)
2. Altered Na^+ or osmotic load in distal tubule detected by distal tubular macula densa which is juxtaposed with JG cells and controls their function. Increased Na^+ or osmotic load inhibits release
3. Increased blood pressure in afferent arteriole → stretching of JG cells → inhibition of renin release.

Factors increasing renin release

Rapid effect factor	*Cause*	*Inhibitor*
Sympathetic stimulation	Lowered BP and/or blood volume Upright posture	β-adrenergic blockers
Adenyl cyclase stimulators	Isoprenaline Noradrenaline Glucagon	β-adrenergic blockers
Vasodilators	Prostaglandins Hydralazine	Vasoconstrictors, e.g. ADH, angiotensin
Diuretics Calcium efflux from JG cells	Frusemide EDTA	β-adrenergic blockers Lanthanum
Slow effect Sodium depletion	Dietary restriction Loss from gut Thiazides Adrenalectomy	Sodium loading Mineralocorticoids

Regulation of the renin-angiotensin system (see Fig. 17.5)

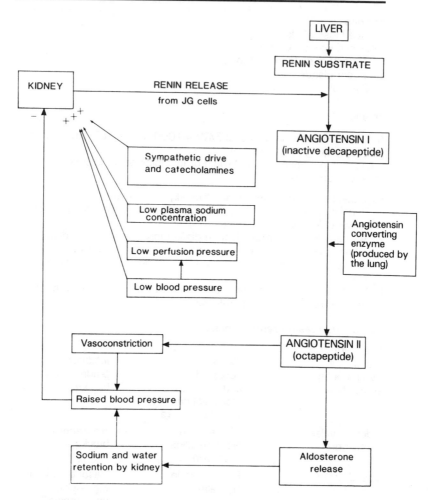

Fig. 17.5 Regulation of the renin-angiotensin system.

Actions of angiotensin II
1. Aldosterone release
2. Powerful vasoconstrictor
   a. Direct Ca^{2+} mediated action
   b. Increased sympathetic tone
3. Other actions
   a. ADH release
   b. Catecholamine release
   c. Thirst centre in CNS activated
   d. CNS-medullary BP centre
   e. Renal Na^+ reabsorption
   f. Smooth muscle contraction—gut and uterus.

Spironolactone
Structural analogue of aldosterone which competes for aldosterone receptors in the distal nephron.

Used mainly to treat oedema in secondary hyperaldosteronism due to excessive release of renin.

Saralasin
1-sarcosyl-8-alanyl-angiotensin II is a specific angiotensin antagonist with some agonist action. It is used diagnostically to detect patients with hypertension due to high renin secretion.

Angiotensin converting enzyme (ACE) inhibitors

Captopril and *Enalapril* are ACE inhibitors, i.e. the conversion angiotensin I $\rightarrow$ angiotensin II is blocked. Thus the vasoconstrictor and aldosterone releasing effects of angiotensin II are antagonised. The drugs are effective hypotensive agents in all forms of hypertension (i.e. low or high renin; low or high aldosterone types). Also valuable to lower peripheral vascular resistance in heart failure.

Toxicity includes rashes, loss of taste, bone marrow depression (large doses) and raised blood potassium (due to reduction in aldosterone secretion). First dose may precipitate marked hypotension especially if combined with diuretics. Can also cause abrupt loss of renal perfusion when renal blood flow is already compromised by renal artery narrowing.

ADRENAL MEDULLA

1. Dopamine uptake
2. Conversion of dopamine $\rightarrow$ noradrenaline
3. Storage of noradrenaline and adrenaline
4. Protection of catecholamines from MAO degradation
5. Release of noradrenaline and adrenaline in response to nerve stimulation. Ca^{2+} is also involved in this.

Conversion of noradrenaline to adrenaline takes place in the cytoplasm (corticosteroid may be involved in this reaction) and the adrenaline is then taken up by the granules.

Release is mediated by nicotinic cholinergic receptors in the adrenal following stimulation of the splanchnic sympathetic nerves, i.e. the adrenal medulla is analogous to a postganglionic sympathetic neurone. (See Ch. 6)

Uses
Uses of adrenaline or analogues, depending on their effects on α or β receptors:
1. Cardiac arrest—to increase myocardial contractility and heart rate (β_1 effects)
2. Hypotension—to increase peripheral vascular resistance (α effect)
3. Anaphylaxis—to relieve bronchospasm (β_2 effect).

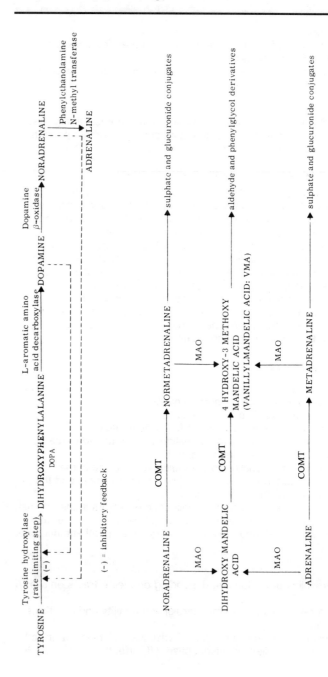

Fig. 17.6 Synthesis and metabolism of catecholamines.

INSULIN

Secreted (with C-chain and proinsulin) from β cells of islets of Langerhans.

Secretion stimulated by:
1. Carbohydrate
   a. Glucose
   b. Fructose
   c. Mannose
2. Free fatty acids
3. Amino acids
4. Raised cAMP
   a. β agonists
   b. Aminophylline
5. Hormones
   a. Glucagon
   b. ACTH
   c. Thyroxine
   d. Growth hormone
   e. Secretin
   f. Gastrin
   g. Pancreozymin
   h. Oestrogens
   i. Placental lactogen
   j. Oestrogens.

Inhibitors of insulin secretion
1. Hypoglycaemia
2. Insulin
3. α agonists
4. β blockers
4. Diazoxide.

Actions
Insulin binds to a specific membrane receptor, this may result in decrease in cellular cAMP and/or increase in cGMP.

Observable effects:
1. Enhanced facilitated diffusion of glucose into cells and increased utilisation of glucose
2. Enhanced active uptake of amino acids and accelerated protein synthesis
3. Accelerated K^+ and Mg^{2+} uptake into cells
4. Fat is formed from pyruvate (due to activation of pyruvate dehydrogenase and lipoprotein lipase)
5. Increased glycogen synthesis (due to reduced sensitivity of protein kinase to cAMP and activation of glycogen synthetase)

Table 17.6 Properties of some insulin preparations

Name of preparation	Action	Peak activity (h)	Duration of action (h)	Source of insulin	Comments
SOLUBLE INSULIN					
SOLUBLE INSULIN	Short	2–4	6–12	Beef	
ISOPHANE INSULIN	Intermediate	3–6	12–16	Beef	
INSULIN ZINC SUSPENSIONS					
Amorphous (Semilente)	Intermediate	3–6	12–16	Pig	
Crystalline (Ultralente)	Short	6–12	24–30	Beef	
Lente	Intermediate	3–8	24–30	30% pig and 70% beef	
MONOCOMPONENT INSULINS					
Actrapid MC	Short	2–4	6–12	Pig	Virtually non antigenic
Monotard	Intermediate	2–5	16–24	Pig	Virtually non antigenic
Semitard	Long	6–10	24–30	Pig	Virtually non antigenic
HUMAN INSULINS					
Human Actrapid (emp)	Short	2–4	6–12	Modified porcine	Theoretically should be less antigenic than all other forms
Humulin S (crb)	Short	2–4	6–12	Bacterial recombinant	

[Humulin Zn (crb), Humulin I (crb) and Human Protophane (emp) are intermediate-long acting human insulins]

emp = enzyme modified porcine
crb = chain recombinant bacterial

6. Decreased catabolism of protein, fat and glycogen (due to stabilisation of lysosomes and dephosphorylation of triglyceride lipase and phosphorylase respectively).

In diabetes insulin produces:
1. Lowering of blood glucose
2. Increased storage of glycogen and fat
3. Reduction in gluconeogenesis
4. Reduction of hyperlipidaemia
5. Abolition of ketosis.

INSULIN EFFECTS

Anticatabolic effects

Liver	*Muscle*	*Fat*
↓ glycogenolysis	↓ protein breakdown	↓ lipolysis
↓ gluconeogenesis	↓ amino acid output	
↓ ketogenesis		

Anabolic effects

↑ glycogen synthesis	↑ amino acid uptake	↓ glycerol synthesis
↑ fatty acid synthesis	↑ protein synthesis	↓ fatty acid synthesis
	↑ glycogen synthesis	

Table 17.7 Classification of diabetes mellitus

	Insulin dependent	*Non-insulin dependent*
	Type I	Type II
Previously known	Juvenile	Maturity onset
Typical patient	Weight loss	Obese
Cause	Insulin deficiency	Insulin resistance
Treatment	Insulin	Diet
		Oral hypoglycaemics

ORAL HYPOGLYCAEMIC AGENTS

1. Sulphonamides
2. Biguanides.

ACTIONS OF SULPHONYLUREAS

1. Islet β cells stimulated to degranulate and secrete more insulin (drugs ineffective in pancreatectomised patients)—imitates and/or enhances response of β cell to glucose. Hypoglycaemia can be produced in normal (and diabetic) individuals
2. Minor effects:
   a. Inhibition of insulin uptake by liver
   b. Enhances antilipolytic action of insulin
3. No effect on glucagon secretion.

ACTIONS OF BIGUANIDES

Hypoglycaemia not readily produced in normal individuals.
No degranulation of islet β cells.
Possible mechanism:
1. Increased peripheral glucose utilisation by enhanced anaerobic glycolysis. Lactate levels rise, dangerous lactic acidosis occurs
2. Decreased gluconeogenesis
3. Inhibition of intestinal absorption of glucose (and vitamin B_{12}).

Examples

Sulphonylureas
  Short acting: gliclazide, gliquidone, tolbutamide
  Long acting: glibenclamide, chlorpropamide (beware hypoglycaemia, especially elderly)
Biguanides
  Short acting: metformin (beware lactic acidosis, especially in renal failure)

Table 17.8 Pharmacokinetic properties of some oral hypoglycaemic agents

Drug	Metabolism and elimination	$t_{1/2}$ (h)	Duration of action (h)
SULPHONYLUREAS			
Tolbutamide	Oxidised in liver, excreted in urine.	4–5	6–12
Chlorpropamide	Minimal metabolism, primarily excreted unchanged in urine.	36	60
Glibenclamide	95% metabolism to inactive hydroxylated metabolites excreted in urine and bile.	5	12
Glipizide	85% metabolism to several inactive hydroxylated metabolites.	2.5–4	6–10
BIGUANIDE			
Metformin	Excreted virtually unchanged in urine.	2–5.5	8–12

18. Lipid-lowering drugs and water-soluble vitamins

LIPOPROTEINS AND DRUG TREATMENT

In patients with hypercholesterolaemia, lowering low density lipoproteins (LDL) and raising high density lipoproteins (HDL) slows the progression of atherosclerosis. Drugs are only used if diet has failed to lower LDL.

HDL cholesterol levels are raised by:
1. Exercise
2. Fish oils
3. Alcohol
4. Nicotinic acid group
5. Clofibrate group.

LDL cholesterol is lowered by:
1. Anion exchange resins
2. Clofibrate group
3. Probucol
4. Nicotinic acid group
5. HMG CoA reductase inhibitors.

Table 18.1 Actions of some lipid-lowering drugs

Drug	Mode of action	Toxicity
RESINS (CHOLESTYRAMINE, COLESTIPOL)	Anion exchange resin which can exchange chloride for bile salt anions. The bound bile salts cannot be absorbed from the gut and the complex is passed in the faeces. As bile salts are lost from the body, more synthesised cholesterol is diverted into the bile salt pool and less enters the circulation. Reduction in bile salt reabsorption also results in increased oxidative removal cholesterol.	Bloating of abdomen. Constipation. Impairs absorption of: vitamins D and K folate phenylbutazone thiazides warfarin antibiotics thyroxin cardiac glycosides.
CLOFIBRATE GROUP (BENZAFIBRATE, FENOFIBRATE, CLOFIBRATE, GEMFIBROZIL)	Decreased synthesis and release of cholesterol by the liver; decreased release of triglycerides into the circulation; increased excretion of neutral sterols (lowers LDL); HDL rises due to mobilisation of tissue cholesterol; decrease in fibrinogen levels; increase in fibrinolysis.	Gallstones Pulmonary emboli Cardiac arrhythmias Nausea Dyspepsia Myositis-like syndrome Rashes Impotence.
NICOTINIC ACID also NICOFURANOSE and ACIPIMOX)	Block off triglyceride synthesis and release by the liver; reduction in synthesis of LDL in patients with type II a, II b and IV hyperlipoproteinaemia.	Itching, flushing, fainting, diarrhoea, nausea, cholestatic jaundice. Hyperuricaemia and gout. Hyperpigmentation.
PROBUCOL	Increases conversion of cholesterol to bile salts.	Diarrhoea, flatulence, nausea, abdominal pain.
HMGCoA REDUCTASE INHIBITORS (SIMVASTATIN and PRAVASTATIN)	Block rate–limiting step in cholesterol synthesis. Lower LDL.	Myositis Gastrointestinal disturbances.
FISH OILS (OMEGA-3 MARINE TRIGLYCERIDES)	Lower triglycerides. Raise HDL. Reduce blood coagulability.	Nausea

Table 18.2 Water-soluble vitamins and their effects

Vitamin	Cellular function	Daily needs	Deficiency states	Hypervitaminosis
Thiamine (vit B_1)	Thiamine pyrophosphate is a coenzyme for decarboxylase—essential for carbohydrate utilisation. Acts at steps of pyruvate and α-ketoglutarate decarboxylation.	Related to calorie intake: 0.4mg/1000 kcals.	Beri–beri: peripheral neuropathy* cardiac failure Alcoholic neuropathy. Wernicke's encephalopathy.** Korsakoff's psychosis.*** Pregnancy neuropathy.	Slight vasodilation on rapid i.v. injection, otherwise no hypervitaminosis state.
Riboflavin (vit B_2)	Converted in body to flavine mononucleotide (FMN) and flavine adenine dinucleotide (FAD). FMN and FAD are coenzymes for a large number of respiratory proteins.	Related to calorie intake: 0.3 mg/1000 kcals (minimum)	Angular stomatitis and sore throat, seborrhoeic dermatitis, itching and burning of eyes, neuropathy, mild anaemia.	No pharmacological actions.
Niacin (Nicotinic acid) and **Nicotinamide** (part of the vit B group)	Converted in body to nicotinamide adenine dinucleotide (NAD) and to NAD phosphate (NADP). Essential in many metabolic steps involving hydrogen transport.	Related to calorie intake: 5 mg niacin/1000 Kcals (minimum). Can be formed from tryptophan—60 mg yields 1 mg of niacin.	Pellagra: light sensitivity dermatitis stomatitis diarrhoea nausea headache depression delusions	Large doses: flushing syncope nausea, vomiting impaired glucose tolerance hyperuricaemia lowers blood lipids

(contd)

Table 18.2 (contd)

Vitamin	Cellular function	Daily needs	Deficiency states	Hypervitaminosis
Several forms of **vitamin B$_6$:** pyridoxine pyridoxal pyridoxamine	Converted in body to pyridoxal phosphate. This is a cofactor in: decarboxylation transamination racemisation.	Related to protein intake: 1.25 mg/100 g Protein (minimal).	Glossitis Seborrhoea Peripheral neuropathy Fits Anaemia.	No pharmacological effects (until very large doses used).
Ascorbic acid (vit C)	Collagen synthesis; steroid metabolism; electron transport and cytochrome P$_{450}$ function; activation of folate; increased gut absorption of iron; hydroxylation of tyrosine, tryptophan, proline.	40–100 mg.	Scurvy: early— malaise weakness lassitude intermediate— dyspnoea bone and joint pains late— perifollicular haemorrhage hyperkeratotic hair follicles skin petechiae and ecchymoses visceral haemorrhages swollen, fragile gums postural hypotension	Large doses can produce hyperoxaluria and urolithiasis.

* Peripheral neuropathy may present as muscle weakness with or without wasting, sensory changes or autonomic disturbances.

** Wernicke's encephalopathy: ocular paralysis, peripheral neuropathy, ataxia, nystagmus, delirium, dementia.

*** Korsakoff's psychosis: severe loss of memory for recent events, confabulation, abnormalities of perception and cognitive function.

19. Drugs acting on the blood

Amongst the factors required for normal erythropoiesis are:
1. Iron
2. Vitamin B_{12}
3. Folic acid.

IRON

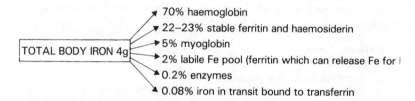

Fig. 19.1

Intestinal absorption of iron:
1. Intestine controls magnitude of iron stores
2. Normal individuals absorb 5–10% of iron in food and in iron salts (more is absorbed by iron deficient patients)
3. Ferrous salts absorbed better than ferric
4. Bulky food, tetracyclines, phytates and phosphate impair absorption
5. Vitamin C, intrinsic factor, alcohol and gastric acid enhance absorption.

Oral iron for iron deficiency anaemia
Ferrous sulphate, gluconate and fumarate:
1. Reticulocyte response starts after 5 days and lasts for 10 days
2. Hb starts to rise at end of 1st week at a rate of 0.1–0.2 g/100 ml blood/d until optimal response reached.

Parenteral iron
Iron dextran (Imferon), iron sorbitol citric acid (Jectofer), and saccharated iron oxide (Ferrivenin).

Toxic effects of parenteral iron:
1. Staining of skin
2. Fever
3. Headache
4. Vomiting
5. Arthralgia
6. Urticaria
7. Lymph node swelling.

VITAMIN B$_{12}$

Vitamin B$_{12}$ = nucleotide + cobalt + 4 pyrrol rings.
Several interconvertible forms of vit B$_{12}$
Cobalt attached to:
1. OH group—hydroxycobalamin
2. Cyanide—cyanocobalamin
3. Methyl—methylcobalamin
4. 5—deoxyadenosyl group.
Normal body stores = 3 mg (takes 3–5 years for depletion). Vit B$_{12}$ absorbed from the lower ileum only when combined with intrinsic factor.

Intrinsic factor
1. Glycoprotein, MW 55 000
2. Secreted by gastric parietal cells
3. Secretion stimulated by histamine and pentagastrin
4. Forms an acid stable complex with vit B$_{12}$.

Actions of vitamin B$_{12}$
1. Erythropoiesis and maturation of other cell types—lack of B$_{12}$ results in a macrocytic anaemia with a megaloblastic bone marrow
2. Isomerisation of methylmalonyl CoA to succinyl CoA
3. Conversion of homocysteine to methionine utilising 5-methyltetrahydrofolate as 1C donor
4. Facilitation of entry of folate into cells (perhaps mechanism of 1).

Administered
By injection for B$_{12}$ deficiency due to:
1. Nutritional lack
2. Failure of absorption (e.g. lack of intrinsic factor as in pernicious anaemia or following gastrectomy)
3. Intestinal disease (e.g. jejunal diverticulosis, Crohn's disease, *Dibothriocephalus latus* infestation).
Usual form given is hydroxycobalamin because:
1. Retained more efficiently
2. Dispersed from injection site more slowly
3. More effectively stored in liver.

The earliest index of a favourable response is a reticulocyte peak at 5 days.

FOLIC ACID

FOLIC ACID = pteridine + p-aminobenzoic acid + glutamate.

Function
After activation, acts as a carrier of 1C fragments including:
1. Methylation of deoxyuridylic acid to form thymidylic acid
2. Other steps in purine and pyrimidine synthesis necessary for normal erythropoiesis: lack produces a macrocytic anaemia with a megaloblastic bone marrow.

Body stores = 70 mg of which one-third is in liver. Stores last about 4 months.

Administered orally for folate deficiency states:
1. Dietary lack
2. Malabsorption
3. Excessive utilisation (e.g. pregnancy, chronic haemolytic anaemia) or loss (long-term dialysis)
4. Drugs (e.g. phenytoin, primidone, phenobarbitone, nitrofurantoin).

FIBRINOGEN—FIBRIN

Fibrinolysis

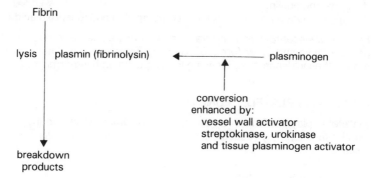

Fig. 19.2

FIBRINOLYTICS
Streptokinase (SK) derived from ultrafiltrates of cultures of Lancefield group C streptococcus haemolyticus.
Urokinase (UK) produced by human fetal kidney cell cultures.
Recombinant tissue plasminogen activator (rt-PA) produced by the cloned human gene in bacteria.

Mode of action
SK—combines with plasminogen in equimolar ratio to form a plasminogen activator complex. Increased circulating plasmin leads to clot lysis.
UK—activates plasminogen directly by cleavage of a single peptide bond.
rt–PA—fibrin specific serine protease that preferentially activates fibrin bound plasminogen compared with plasma fibrinogen.

Use
Effective in coronary thrombosis if used early. Also in portal and hepatic vein thrombosis. Role in uncomplicated deep vein thrombosis in the calf unproven.

Toxicity
SK—hypersensitivity reaction in 15% recipients.
All types may cause bleeding.

ANTIFIBRINOLYTICS
Plasmin formation antagonised by:
   plasminogen activator inhibitor tranexamic acid
Plasmin activity antagonised by:
1. $\alpha_1$antitrypsin
2. $\alpha_1$antiplasmin
3. $\alpha_1$macroglobulin.
Plasmin formation and activity blocked by epsilon aminocaproic acid.

Epsilon aminocaproic acid and tranexamic acid are used to reduce postoperative and other forms of bleeding. Tranexamic acid may reduce the incidence of re-bleeding in subarachnoid haemorrhage.

DRUGS AND PLATELET FUNCTION

Platelets   play a role in thrombus formation. Drugs which modify platelet function may reduce the incidence of occlusive vascular disease.

Drugs which affect platelet function
1. Aspirin:
   Inhibits platelet release reaction and platelet aggregation by inhibiting platelet cyclo–oxygenase and thus blocking production of labile endoperoxides and thromboxane A_2.
2. Sulphinpyrazone:
   Has an antithrombotic action by reducing platelet adherence to vessel wall. Some reduction in platelet aggregation by (weak) inhibition of platelet prostaglandin synthesis.

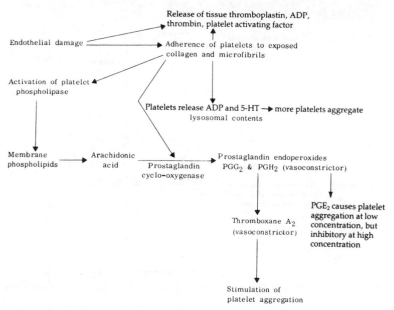

Fig. 19.3

3. Dipyridamole:
   Inhibits platelet release reaction and platelet aggregation, but this has not been demonstrated in man in vivo.
   Inhibits phosphodiesterase: raised platelet cAMP may result in antithrombotic action.

ANTICOAGULANTS

Blood clotting factors:
   I   fibrinogen
   II prothrombin
   III thromboplastin (tissue factor III)
   IV calcium
   V   pro-accelerin
   (VI not used)
   VII proconvertin
   VIII antihaemophilic factor (AHF)
   IX Christmas factor (plasma thromboplastin component (PTC))
   X   Stuart–Prower factor
   XI plasma thromboplastin antecedent (PTA)
   XII Hageman factor (contact factor)
   XIII fibrin stabilising factor.

CLOTTING CASCADE

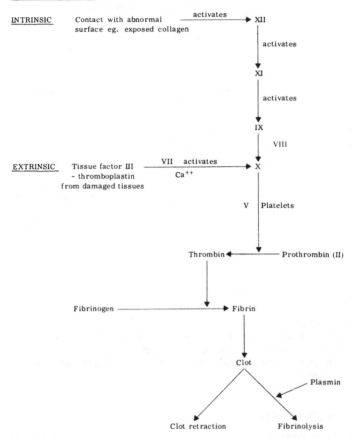

Fig. 19.4

Antithrombin III is a naturally occurring inhibitor of coagulation enzymes:
1. XIIa
2. XIa
3. IXa
4. Xa
5. Thrombin.
Heparin greatly accelerates the action of antithrombin III.

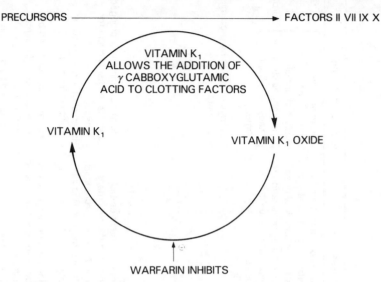

PRECURSORS ─────────────────────────► FACTORS II VII IX X

VITAMIN K₁
ALLOWS THE ADDITION OF
γ CABBOXYGLUTAMIC
ACID TO CLOTTING FACTORS

VITAMIN K₁

VITAMIN K₁ OXIDE

WARFARIN INHIBITS

Fig. 19.5

GROWTH FACTORS

The genes for a number of clinically useful cytokines have been
cloned and by recombinant DNA technology the proteins have been
produced in pharmacological amounts.

RECOMBINANT HUMAN ERYTHROPOIETIN (rHu EPO)

Function
Binds to receptors on early erythroid progenitors in bone marrow.
Increases proliferation and maturation of erythroid precursors leading
to increased red cell production.

Administration
Given intravenously three times per week or subcutaneously twice
weekly. Dose varies according to response. Response depends on
adequate iron stores. Response impaired by iron deficiency or
co-existing infection.

Use
1. To correct the anaemia of chronic renal failure
2. Occasionally helpful in the anaemia of chronic inflammation such as
   rheumatoid arthritis
3. For self donation of blood before major surgery.

Table 19.1 Comparison of three anticoagulants

Anticoagulant	Mode of action	Onset	Clinical uses	Control of therapy
HEPARIN —sulphated acid mucopolysaccharide prepared from beef lung and intestine.	1. Acts as an antithrombin and thus prevents conversion of fibrinogen $\rightarrow$ fibrin*. 2. Inhibition of activated factor X*. 3. Inhibition of activated factor IX. 4. Inhibits the activation of factor IX by XI. Also: Is active in vitro and in vivo; activates lipoprotein lipase; inhibits platelet aggregation by fibrin. (*These actions require the presence of antithrombin III, a plasma factor.)	Immediate.	Continuous or intermittent i.v. administration for arterial and venous thrombosis; low dose subcutaneous administration for prophylaxis of deep vein thrombosis. $t_{1/2}$ = 90min	Thrombin time Clotting time Activated partial thromboplastin time (kaolin–cephalin time) } all prolonged Reversal of action by protamine sulphate.
WARFARIN —a 4-hydroxy-coumarin.	Prevents the reduction of vitamin K_1 oxide to active vitamin K_1. This blocks the synthesis of factors II, VII, IX and X.	Effective after 24—36 h.	Given orally prevent embolic disease and in the treatment of arterial and venous thrombosis. $t_{1/2}$ = 44h (but much individual variation).	Prothrombin time is prolonged and is the usual guide for dose. Reversal of action by water soluble vitamin K.
ANCROD —glycoprotein from the venom of the Malayan pit viper.	Acts as an anticoagulant by destroying fibrinogen. Any fibrin formed is unstable.	Rapid.	Given i.v. for central retinal vein thrombosis, priapism and sickle cell crisis. $t_{1/2}$ = several days.	Treatment is monitored by measurement of plasma fibrinogen. Antagonised by a specific antivenom.

Toxicity
Hypertension due to rapid or excessive rise in haematocrit and increased peripheral vascular resistance.

RECOMBINANT HUMAN GRANULOCYTE STIMULATING FACTOR (rHuG–CSF)

Function
Binds to marrow progenitor cells committed primarily to the production of neutrophils. Increases production and release of neutrophils into the circulation.

Administration
Given subcutaneously once per day or less frequently according to response.

Use
1. Shortens the period of neutropenia following cytotoxic chemotherapy or bone marrow transplantation
2. Increases neutrophil count in myelodysplasia with neutropenia.
3. Increases the neutrophil count in moderate (but not severe) aplastic anaemia.

Toxicity
1. Bone pain
2. Sweet's syndrome (acute febrile neutrophilic dermatosis).

20. Antimicrobial drugs

Antibiotics
Compounds synthesised by micro-organisms which kill or inhibit the growth of the other micro-organisms, e.g. penicillin, streptomycin.

Chemotherapeutic substances
Compounds synthesised in vitro to kill or inhibit growth of micro-organisms in vivo, e.g. sulphonamides.

Bacteriostatic/cidal distinction is relative and probably of little importance under most (but not all) clinical circumstances. In general, *drug combinations* of bactericidal and bacteriostatic drugs may be synergistic, additive or antagonistic.

SULPHONAMIDES

Mode of action
Block bacterial folic acid synthesis by combining with pteridine to form an inactive complex.

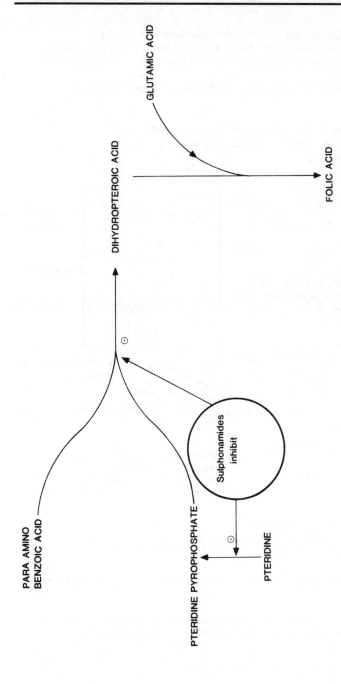

Fig. 20.1 Mode of action of sulphonamides.

Uses

Sulphonamides are currently little used on their own, but combinations with other folate inhibitors (such as co-trimoxazole (sulphamethoxazole plus trimethoprim) are chest and urinary tract infections.

Trimethoprim is also used on its own in urinary infections.

Toxicity

1. Rashes (including Stevens–Johnson syndrome)
2. Highly sensitising when applied topically
3. Dizziness

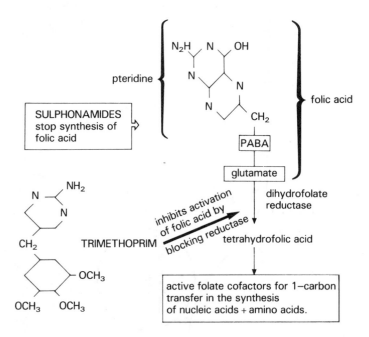

PABA = para amino benzoic acid

SULPHONAMIDES are specifically antibacterial because mammalian cells do not synthesise folic acid but can absorb and utilise the complete molecule. Bacteria have to synthesise the substance intracellularly.

TRIMETHOPRIM acts as a selective antibacterial because it inhibits bacterial dihydrofolate reductase 20 000–60 000 times more powerfully than the mammalian form of the enzyme.

Fig. 20.2 Structural analogy of trimethoprim with pteridine portion of folic acid and its action as an inhibitor of bacterial dihydrofolate reductase.

4. Kernicterus (when given in last 2 weeks of pregnancy or to neonate) because displaces bilirubin from protein binding and bilirubin can then enter and damage brain
5. Haemolytic anaemia (in G6PD deficiency)
6. Crystalluria (especially with sulphadiazine)
7. Aplastic anaemia.

THE PENICILLINS

Penicillinic nucleus + side chains
Nucleus = fused lactam and thiazolidine rings

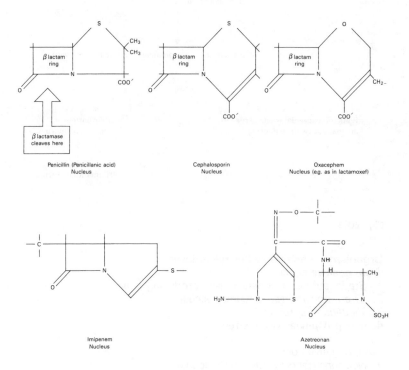

Fig. 20.3 Basic structures of β lactam antibiotics.

Mode of action

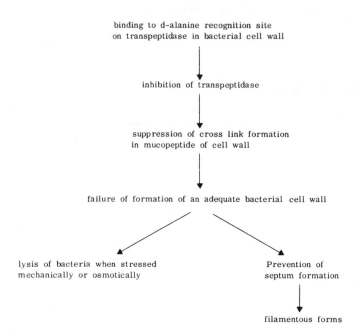

binding to d-alanine recognition site
on transpeptidase in bacterial cell wall

↓

inhibition of transpeptidase

↓

suppression of cross link formation
in mucopeptide of cell wall

↓

failure of formation of an adequate bacterial cell wall

lysis of bacteria when stressed
mechanically or osmotically

Prevention of
septum formation

↓

filamentous forms

Fig. 20.4

Organisms sensitive to benzylpenicillin
Gram positive cocci:
1. *Staph. aureus*—not penicillinase producing strains
2. *Strep. pneumoniae* (pneumococcus)
3. *Viridans streptococci*
4. Group A *β*-haemolytic strep.

Gram negative cocci:
1. *Neisseria gonorrhoeae* (gonococcus)
2. *Neisseria meningitidis* (meningococcus).

Gram positive bacilli:
1. *Bacillus anthracis*
2. *Corynebacterium diphtheriae*
3. *Listeria monocytogenes*
4. Anaerobes including *Clostridium* sp.

Spirochaetes:
1. *T. pallidum* (syphilis)
2. *T. pertenue* (yaws)
3. *Leptospira icterohaemorrhagiae* (Weil's disease).
Actinomyces.

Pencillin toxicity
1. Hypersensitivity:
    Type 1 reactions (early)
    a. Rash (common)—urticaria, erythema
    b. Anaphylaxis (rare)—circulatory collapse, bronchospasm, laryngeal oedema
    Serum sickness (type III reactions)—delayed by 2–12 days: fever, malaise, arthralgia, angioedema, erythema nodosum, exfoliative dermatitis, erythema multiforme, Stevens–Johnson syndrome.

2. Neurotoxicity:
    a. Only high doses (those which may be used with carbenicillin)
    b. Impaired renal function
    c. Intrathecal injection of over 50 000 U
    Encephalopathy can present as:
    a. Fits, coma
    b. Permanent sequelae
    c. Death.

3. Haemolytic anaemia: only high doses.

4. Ampicillin, talampicillin and pivampicillin produce rash (usually morbilliform) in about 8% of patients, more commonly in young women. A very high incidence of this reaction occurs in infectious mononucleosis.

Note: Apart from hypersensitivity, the penicillins are relatively non-toxic and safe drugs.

CEPHALOSPORINS
Similarities to penicillin
1. All cephalosporins have a peptide nucleus (7-amino cephalosporanic acid).
2. Prevent bacterial cell wall formation by inhibiting cross linking in mucopeptide via transpeptidase inhibition similar to penicillin
3. Destroyed by a specific bacterial β-lactamase (cephalosporinase).

Table 20.1 The penicillins

Drug	Administration	Special features	Main uses
Benzylpenicillin (soluble penicillin; penicillin G)	Intramuscularly or intravenously 4–6 hourly	Destroyed by acid and pepsin. Highly bactericidal against susceptible organisms, but destroyed by penicillinase (β-lactamase).	1. Serious infections needing parenteral antibiotic, e.g. meningitis, endocarditis. 2. Infections due to sensitive organisms, e.g. streptococci.
Phenoxymethylpenicillin (Penicillin V)	Oral, 6 hourly.	Resistant to acid hydrolysis—same properties as benzylpenicillin.	All main uses of benzylpenicillin apart from most serious infections.
Flucloxacillin	Oral, 6 hourly	Resistant to attack by staphylococcal β lactamase (as are cloxacillin and methicillin).	Staphylococcal infections—including penicillinase producing organisms.
Ampicillin	Oral, 6 hourly	Resistant to acid hydrolysis but destroyed by β lactamase. Inhibits end wall synthesis of bacterial cell. Effective against Gram negative organisms which are not susceptible to benzylpenicillin—e.g. coliforms and *Haemophilus influenzae*, but 50% of coliforms are now resistant.	Gram negative infections of the respiratory and urinary tracts. Otitis media.
Talampicillin and Pivampicillin	Oral, 8 hourly.	Ampicillin prodrugs: hydrolysed in the intestinal mucosa to ampicillin.	As ampicillin. ? any advantage over ampicillin.
Amoxycillin	Oral, 8 hourly.	Derivative of ampicillin which differs by only one OH group. Similar spectrum but (a) better absorbed when given by mouth achieving higher plasma and tissue levels (b) more effective against Salmonella.	As ampicillin plus prophylaxis of bacterial endocarditis.

Carbenicillin	Intravenous infusions with high doses.	Not absorbed from gut. Similar broad spectrum as ampicillin, but effective against *Ps. aeruginosa* and *Proteus* spp.	Mainly reserved for serious pseudomonas and proteus infections.
Pivmecillinam —prodrug of mecillinam	Oral, 6–8 hourly.	Hydrolysed during absorption to mecillinam. One of a group of amidinopenicillins—an amidino group replaces the NH_2 group at position 6 of the penicillin nucleus. This greatly increases activity against Gram negative organisms (and decreases action on Gram positive organisms). Destroyed by some, but not all, types of β-lactamase.	Gram negative infections (including Salmonellae) resistant to ampicillin.
Mezlocillin azlocillin abd piperacillin	Injected	Ureidopenicillins, active against Gram-negative bacilli, some staphylococci and many anaerobes	Treatment and prophylaxis of intestinal, biliary, urinary and blood borne infections.

N.B. Clavulanic acid is a β-lactamase inhibitor. It is combined with amoxycillin in Augmentin, which is resistant to β-lactamase.

CLASSIFICATION

At present the cephalosporins are grouped on a historical basis:

First generation
1. Oral (e.g. cephradine; cefaclor). Used in respiratory and urinary infections. Little activity against haemophilus but many staphylococci are sensitive
2. Parenteral (e.g. cephaloridine; cephalothin). Inactivated by β-lactamases from Gram-negative bacilli.

Second generation
(e.g. cefuroxime; cefamandole; cefoxitin). All injected but oral cefuroxime now available as cefuroxime axetil. Effective against staphylococci, streptocci and Gram negative bacteria (including *E coli*, *Proteus* spp, *Klebsiella* spp, *H. Influenzae* and *N. gonorrhoeae*). Relatively resistant to β-lactamases.

Third generation
All injected
1. Cefotaxime: effective against most Gram-negative bacilli (but weak activity against pseudomonas). *H. influenzae* and *N. gonorrhoeae* very sensitive
2. Latamoxef: similar spectrum to cefotaxime, but more effective against anaerobes including. *B. fragilis*
   Both cefotaxime and latamoxef used in speticaemia, meningitis and other serious infections due to *E. coli*
3. Cefsulodin: mainly active against *P. aeruginosa*
4. Ceftazidime: Effective against *P. aeruginosa* and other Gram-negative bacilli.

Features common to all the cephalosporins
1. Mainly excreted via kidneys
2. Do not penetrate well into sputum
3. Used mainly for penicillin resistant staphylococcal infections, urinary tract infections, syphillis and gonorrhoea
   Less often for soft tissue and respiratory infections
4. Allergic rashes occur—10% of patients sensitive to penicillin react to cephalosporins.

ERYTHROMYCIN

Description
A member of the macrolide group—all of which have a lactone ring linked to sugar molecules. Other members, such as oleandomycin and spiramycin, have similar but weaker antibacterial properties.

Table 20.2 Antibiotics which act on bacterial ribosomes

Antibiotic	Main ribosomal component involved	Mode of action	Resistance
AMINOGLYCOSIDES	30S	Bind to specific protein on 30S subunit and freeze initiation complexes; also produce misreading of mRNA code.	Mutation of binding protein in 30S subunit; also an antibiotic inactivated by phosphorylation, adenylation and acetylation.
TETRACYLINES	30S	Susceptible organisms concentrate tetracycline intracellularly; both 30S and 50S subunits are bound and tetracyclines prevent tRNA binding to A site.	New protein in 30S subunit which prevents active uptake of drug.
CHLORAMPHENICOL	50S	Binds and distorts 50S subunits and thus prevents transpeptidation.	Production of enzymes which acetylate chloramphenicol.
ERYTHROMYCIN	50S	Prevents translocation by binding to 50S subunit.	Change in protein or RNA in 50S subunit which prevents binding.
FUSIDIC ACID	50S	Inhibits translocation of tRNA; blocks availability of energy and factor G to do this: cell wall collapses because of lack of protein	
CLINDAMYCIN	50S	Similar to erythromycin which competes with it.	

BACTERIAL RIBOSOMES CONTAIN 30s & 50s SUBUNITS
A SITE = acceptor site
P SITE = peptidyl synthetase enzyme

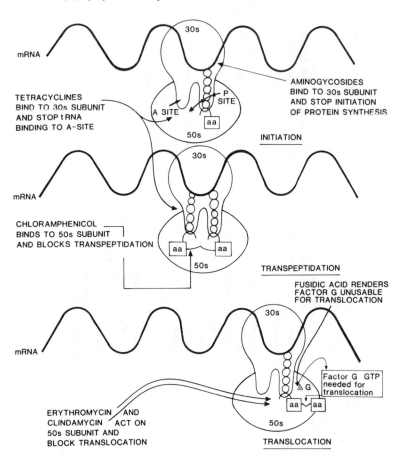

Fig. 20.5 The sites of action of antibacterials on ribosomes.

Inhibition of bacterial ribosome protein synthesis by block of peptide translocase on the 50s ribosome subunit.

Pharmacokinetics

Erythromycin base is destroyed by gastric acid, but the estolate and palmitate are given orally. Little enters CSF. Mainly metabolised, $t_{1/2}$ = 1.5—3h.

Antibacterial activity
Bacteriostatic for β-haemolytic streptococci, *Staphylococcus aureus*, Neisseria, *H. influenzae, Mycoplasma pneumoniae, Legionella pneumophila* and *E. coli*.

Uses
1. Alternative drug for patients allergic to penicillin—particularly for streptococcal, pneumococcal and gonococcal infections
2. Mycoplasma pneumonia
3. Diphtheria carriers
4. Legionnaires' disease.

Toxicity
Erythromycin base is not toxic. The estolate can produce hepatitis–like syndrome (pain, jaundice, eosinophilia, cholestasis). Also: GI disturbances, allergy.

CHLORAMPHENICOL

Description
1. Broad spectrum antibiotic. Bacteriostatic
2. Simple nitrobenzene derivative.

Mode of action
1. Inhibits bacterial 70 S ribosomes at the 50 S subunit and blocks peptidyl transferase
2. Can also block function of animal mitochondrial 70 S ribosomes— but cannot usually pass through mitochondrial membrane.

Pharmacokinetics
Well absorbed from intestine and injection sites. Penetrates very well throughout body water—enters CSF. Excreted after reduction or glucuronidation. Metabolism reduced in immature neonatal liver, hence toxicity occurs.

Activity and use
Wide range of Gram–positive and negative organisms susceptible but because of toxicity use is restricted to serious infections by Salmonellae (e.g. typhoid), *H. influenzae* and organisms resistant to other drugs.

Toxicity
Marrow aplasia (rare but important because usually fatal—idiosyncratic). Marrow depression (reversible, dose dependent). Sore mouth, nausea, diarrhoea, grey baby syndrome in neonate (a condition of circulatory collapse), optic neuritis.

Table 20.3 Tetracycline drugs

Drug	Special features	Use
TETRACYCLINE OXYTETRACYCLINE	Cheapest and most widely used of group. Subject to variation in intestinal absorption—particularly inhibited by Ca^{2+} in food.	All main indications for tetracyclines.
CHLORTETRACYCLINE	Probably more prone to produce gastrointestinal disturbances when given by mouth.	Applied locally (e.g. to conjunctiva, ear) but can produce sensitisation.
DEMECLOCYCLINE	Better intestinal absorption than the above.	Inappropriate secretion of ADH (blocks effect of hormone on renal tubule).
DOXYCYCLINE	The only tetracycline which is safe in renal failure because excreted in bile. Well absorbed—even if food in stomach. Prolonged $t_{1/2}$. Enters sinuses and middle ear fluids well.	Infections in patients with renal failure. Sinusitis. Middle ear infections. Prophylaxis 'travellers diarrhoea'.
MINOCYCLINE	Active against meningococci. Well absorbed even if food is in stomach. Can cause vertigo.	Treating sulphonamide resistant meningococci in carriers. Non-specific urethritis. Respiratory and urinary tract infections.

NB Tetracyclines can all produce photosensitive rashes although some, e.g. demeclocycline, are more liable to do this than others.

TETRACYCLINES

Mode of action
1. Acts on 80 S (animal) and 70 S (bacterial) ribosomes and inhibits protein synthesis
2. Bacteriostatic (not bacteriocidal) therefore not drugs of choice in endocarditis or leucopenia.

Kinetics
Usually well absorbed from gut, but chelate with Fe, Al and Ca and therefore food blocks absorption. Penetrate into body fluids—including sputum. Renal excretion.

Toxicity
1. Diarrhoea common
2. Monilial super-infections
3. Aggravation of uraemia—anti-anabolic effect
4. Staining of teeth if exposed to drug in fetal life or childhood
5. Interfere with absorption of oral iron.

Spectrum and uses (see Table 20.3)
Broad spectrum but proteus, pseudomonas and many staphylococci and streptococci are resistant.
Main uses:
1. Exacerbation of bronchitis (haemophilus and *Strep. pneumoniae*, but resistance appearing)
2. Psittacosis, Q fever, typhus, trachoma and inclusion conjunctivitis (chlamydial)
3. *Mycoplasma pneumoniae*
4. Nonspecific urethritis and lymphogranuloma venereum
5. Brucellosis
6. Acne
7. Syphilis, anthrax and actinomycosis in patients allergic to penicillin
8. Cholera.

CLINDAMYCIN

Acts similarly to erythromycin on bacterial ribosome function and therefore competes with it. Well absorbed by mouth and penetrates tissues (including bone) well, but not CSF. Limited use because of toxicity—rare but fatal pseudomembranous colitis due to *Clostridium difficile* toxin, which is sensitive to vancomycin and metronidazole by mouth. Main use is for staphylococcal bone infections and bacteroides (and other anaerobes) when other antibiotics cannot be used.

AMINOGLYCOSIDES

The aminoglycosides are produced by Streptomyces spp. and Microsporum spp. Effective against many Gram—negative bacilli. Also show clinically useful synergy with penicillins against some streptococci. Inactive against anaerobes.

Table 20.4 Aminoglycosides: individual drugs

Drug	Special features	Clinical uses
STREPTOMYCIN	Prone to ototoxicity and thus avoid in the elderly and in patients with renal failure. Inactive against *Ps. aeruginosa*.	Rarely used—now a second line drug in TB. Effective against some strains of *Staph. aureus*, *E. coli* and *H. influenzae*.
KANAMYCIN	Both ototoxic (cochlea) and nephrotoxic. Not effective against *Ps. aeruginosa*.	Some Gram negative septicaemias. May be used to treat TB and gonorrhoea resistant to more usual drugs. Mainly superceded by gentamicin.
NEOMYCIN	Too toxic for systemic use. Local use encourages emergence of resistant strains. Local sensitivity.	Topical application and intestinal sterilisation.
GENTAMICIN	Broad antibacterial spectrum including *Ps. aeruginosa*, staphylococci and coliforms. Ototoxicity (vestibular) and nephrotoxicity can be prevented by attention to blood levels.	Important drug in the treatment of life-threatening infections: septicaemia, pyelonephritis, cholangitis, surgical sepsis and sepsis in the newborn and immunosuppressed patients due to Gram-negative bacilli (including pseudomonas).
TOBRAMYCIN	Similar spectrum and toxicity to gentamicin but 2-4 times more active against *Ps. aeruginosa*. Complete cross-resistance.	Same as for gentamicin.
AMIKACIN	Ototoxic (cochlea). Semisynthetic derivative of kanamycin. The introduction of a side chain protects the molecule against enzymic attack which is the basis of bacterial resistance to the aminoglycosides. This confers a particularly wide spectrum of activity.	Reserved for major coliform and pseudomonas infections resistant to gentamicin. Can be used in combined therapy for TB resistant to streptomycin.
NETILMYCIN	Similar activity to gentamycin but effective against a number of gentamicin-resistant strains and less active against *Ps. aeruginosa*. Less ototoxic.	Severe Gram-negative infections resistant to gentamicin.

Mode of action
Powerful bactericidal action. Bind to a specific protein in the 30 S subunit of bacterial ribosomes blocking bacterial ribosomal protein synthesis by interfering with initiation complex. Also causes misreading of mRNA. Do not bind to human ribosomes.

Pharmacokinetics
1. Very little intestinal absorption. However, in renal failure enough may accumulate in plasma to result in toxicity
2. Excreted in active form via glomerular filtrate by kidneys. Thus plasma levels must be monitored in all patients, particularly those with renal failure. 25–50% of plasma concentration in pleural fluid, sputum, bile, joint and peritoneal fluid
3. Much less penetrates into CSF.

Toxicity
1. Ototoxic—auditory and vestibular functions of VIII cranial nerve
2. Nephrotoxic
3. Block of motor end plate potentiates the action of curare-like drugs
4. Allergy—contact dermatitis (common), drug fever, rash (uncommon).

Bacterial resistance
This is common and can appear rapidly.
Resistance can be acquired from other organisms by transmission of plasmids.
These allow organisms to synthesise:
1. Inactivating enzymes
   a. Acetylases
   b. Adenylases
   c. Phosphorylases
2. Permeability factors which prevent antibiotic penetration.

VANCOMYCIN AND TEICOPLANIN
1. These are bactericidal glycopeptide antibiotics derived from *Nocardia orientalis* and *Actinoplanes teicomyceticus* respectively
2. They act by inhibiting bacterial cell wall synthesis
3. Always given parenterally. Relatively long $\frac{1}{2}$-life (12h for vancomycin; 24h for teicoplanin)
4. Toxicity: ototoxic and nephrotoxic; plasma concentration should be monitored especially in patients with renal impairment
5. Used for multiply-resistant staphylococci and other Gram + ve cocci. Given by mouth for pseudomembranous colitis.

AZTREONAM
1. Monocyclic β-lactam active against aerobic Gram – ve bacteria

2. Toxicity includes hypersensitivity to other β-lactam antibiotics (Fig. 20.3), gastrointestinal disturbance, bone marrow depression, hepatitis
3. Used against *Pseudomonas aeruginosa* and *neisseria.*

IMIPENAM
1. The first thienamycin β-lactam antibiotic
2. Partially inactivated by an enzyme in the kidney. Therefore given with cilastin (which inhibits this enzyme)
3. Cross hypersensitivity with other β-lactams. Neurotoxicity in renally impaired patients
4. Broad spectrum against Gram + ve and − ve bacteria.

4-QUINOLONES
Antibacterials chemically related to nalidixic acid. The latter is relatively toxic, but ciprofloxacin, enoxacin and ofloxacin are useful, particularly for urinary infections. Acrosoxacin is used for gonorrhoea. Ciprofloxacin is also used for systemic and respiratory tract infections.

The quinolones have little useful action against Gram + ve cocci. They act by inhibiting bacterial DNA gyrase, an enzyme not present in mammalian tissues.

The 4-quinolones may lower brain GABA and thus predispose to fits.

FUSIDIC ACID (FUCIDIN)
A relatively non-toxic, steroidal antibiotic, reserved for the treatment of staphylococcal infections especially osteomyelitis. Inhibits bacterial ribosome translocase by binding to 50S subunit and preventing release and reuse of factor G.

NITROFURANTOIN
1. A nitrofuran used solely in the treatment of urinary tract infections
2. Blocks bacterial carbohydrate metabolism by inhibition of acetyl CoA synthesis. 30% appears in urine unmetabolised
3. Toxicity (nausea and peripheral neuropathy) likely in renal dysfunction
4. Contraindicated in renal failure.

SPECTINOMYCIN
1. Aminocyclitol antibiotic with broad spectrum. It acts of the 30S subunit in a way similar to the aminoglycosides but does not cause misreading of mRNA
2. Used in man only for gonorrhoea—it has no effect on concomitant syphilis
3. Given by injection only.

METRONIDAZOLE

Description
Synthetic, heterocyclic nitro derivative.

Mode of action
1. Blocks energy production from carbohydrates by inhibiting a reductase in Clostridia and other anaerobes. Inhibits anaerobic electron transfer chain
2. Specific to anaerobic organisms because it must be reduced to an active derivative which binds to DNA and blocks nucleic axid synthesis.

Pharmacokinetics
Absorbed orally and rectally. Can be given i.v. Enters abscess fluid. $t_{1/2}$ = 6–8 h. 70% excreted unchanged in urine but usually no cumulation in renal failure.

Activity and use
Active against anaerobic micro-organisms only. Used in *Trichomonas vaginalis* and *Giardia lamblia* infections; acute ulcerative stomatitis, amoebic dysentery and abscess; anaerobic infections due to *Bacteroides fragilis*, Fusobacteria, Clostridia, anaerobic streptococci and Eubacteria; Guinea worm; tropical ulcer.

Toxicity
Metallic taste (due to salivary excretion of drug). GI disturbances, rashes, drowsiness, antabuse-like reaction with alcohol; peripheral neuropathy after large doses used for a long time.

DRUGS USED IN THE TREATMENT OF TUBERCULOSIS

First line drugs
1. Isoniazid (INH; isonicotinic acid hydrazide)
2. Ethambutol
3. Rifampicin
4. Pyrazinamide.

Second line drugs (used if TB relapses after previous treatment)
1. Streptomycin
2. PAS (para-aminosalicylic acid)
3. Cycloserine
4. Capreomycin
5. Kanamycin.

The initial phase of treatment lasts at least 8 weeks. In this, at least three drugs are given to prevent the emergence of resistance— isoniazid with rifampicin supplemented with ethambutol, usually with the further addition of pyrazinamide. The continuation phase

Table 20.5 First line antituberculous drugs

Drug	Pharmacokinetics	Activity	Toxicity
ISONIAZID (INH)	Good intestinal absorption. Penetrates into all body fluids including CSF and enters macrophages. Genetically determined speed of acetylation. $t_{1/2} < 80$ mins in rapid acetylators; $t_{1/2} > 140$ mins in slow acetylators.	Powerfully anti-TB. Inhibits formation of mycolic acid in bacterial cell wall.	Insomnia, muscle twitching, peripheral neuropathy (responds to vitamin B_6), hepatitis-like syndrome.
ETHAMBUTOL	Good intestinal absorption. Concentrated in r.b.c.'s which act as reservoir. 80% excreted unchanged in urine— contraindicated in renal dysfunction. $t_{1/2} = 5$–6 h.	Concentrated in tubercle bacilli, but mode of action not known. Resistance develops slowly. Effective against strains resistant to INH and streptomycin.	In high doses: retrobulbar neuritis (green vision lost first), rashes, pruritus, joint pains, nausea, abdominal pain, confusion, hallucinations, peripheral neuropathy.
RIFAMPICIN	Complete absorption from intestine. Penetrates into all body fluids except CSF. Enters macrophages. Majority is metabolised and excreted in bile. Usually no cumulation in renal dysfunction. $t_{1/2} = 1.5$–5 h. Powerful enzyme inducer.	Inhibits RNA polymerase in bacteria. Resistance can develop rapidly if used on its own.	Flu-like illness, hepatotoxic, thrombocytopenia (rare), rashes, pink urine.
PYRAZINAMIDE	Absorbed from intestine. Renal excretion. Enters macrophages.	Bacteriostatic in acid environment. Inhibits growth of tubercle bacilli in monocytes.	Hepatotoxic. Can precipitate gout. Fever.

consists of administering two drugs one of which is isoniazid.
Treatment lasts a minimum of 6 months in total depending on the
combination used.

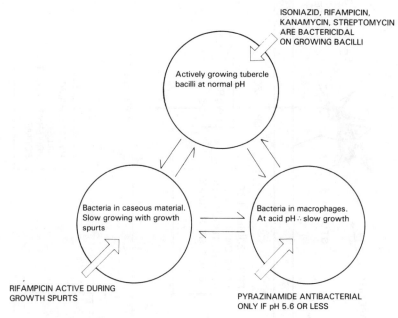

ISONIAZID, RIFAMPICIN,
KANAMYCIN, STREPTOMYCIN
ARE BACTERICIDAL
ON GROWING BACILLI

Actively growing tubercle
bacilli at normal pH

Bacteria in caseous material.
Slow growing with growth
spurts

Bacteria in macrophages.
At acid pH ∴ slow growth

RIFAMPICIN ACTIVE DURING
GROWTH SPURTS

PYRAZINAMIDE ANTIBACTERIAL
ONLY IF pH 5.6 OR LESS

Fig. 20.6 Site of action of anti-TB drugs.

ANTIMALARIALS

Prophylaxis*
1. 4-amino quinolines: chloroquine
                                   amodiaquine
2. Dihydrofolate reductase inhibitors: pyrimethamine
                                                        proguanil

Prophylaxis of chloroquine-resistant malaria
1. Dapsone with proguanil
2. Maloprim (pyrimethamine with dapsone)
3. Fansidar (pyrimethamine with sulphadoxine).

Drugs used in treatment of acute attack*
1. Chloroquine
2. Quinine.

*Reference centres should be consulted for the most recent information on
antimalarial resistance patterns.

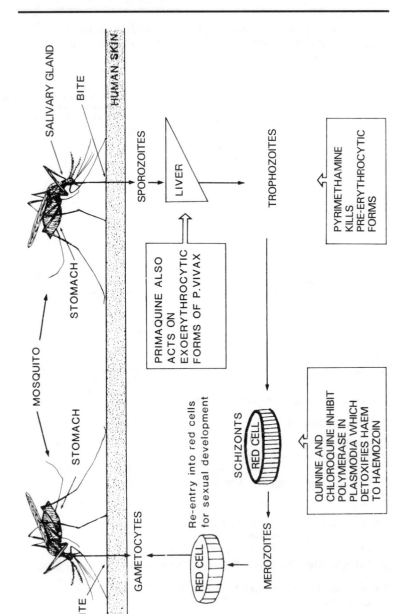

Fig. 20.7 Sites of action of drugs on life cycle of malarial parasite.

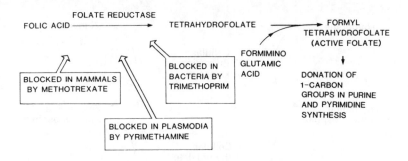

Fig. 20.8 Site of action of pyrimethamine in plasmodia.

ANTIVIRAL DRUGS

Specific targets
1. Viral penetration and uncoating:
   Blocked by *amantadine* and *rimantadine*
   Used in influenza A prophylaxis
2. Viral specific enzymes:
   a. *Acyclovir* (related to guanosine) is phosphorylated 30–120 times faster by virus-induced thymidine kinase than by host enzyme to form acyclo guanosine triphosphate. This inhibits herpes specific DNA polymerase 10–30 times more than cellular DNA polymerase. Also acyclovir inhibits DNA synthesis by acting as a substrate and when incorporated into DNA terminates synthesis. Used in severe herpes simplex or herpes zoster infections
   b. *Gancyclovir* related to acyclovir but with enhanced toxicity against cytomegalovirus. It causes bone marrow suppression and is only indicated for prevention or suppression of life-threatening infection in immunocompromised hosts
   c. *Vidarabine* inhibits herpes-specific DNA polymerase by forming hypoxanthine arabinoside
   d. *Idoxuridine* substitutes in viral DNA in place of thymidine. In this way stops replication of viral DNA. Used for local treatment of herpes simplex and zoster
   e. *Zidovudine (AZT)* phosphorylated by thymidine kinase in virally-infected and non-infected cells. Further phosphorylated to zidovudine triphosphate which is the active form. Blocks the synthesis of pro-viral DNA by viral reverse transcriptase. Active against retroviruses and used to treat patients with advanced HIV disease. Causes myelotoxicity and gastrointestinal symptoms

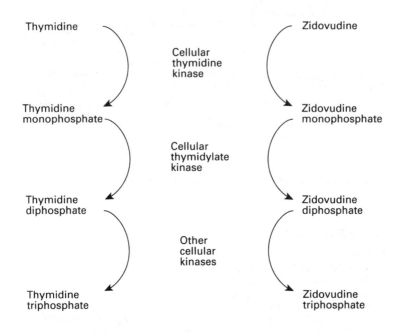

Fig. 20.9 Phosphorylation of zidovudine and thymidine to their triphosphates. Zidovudine triphosphate interferes with pro-viral DNA synthesis by (1) competition with thymidine triphosphate for binding sites on the enzyme reverse transcriptase (2) incorporation into and termination of the pro-viral DNA chain.

3. Translation of viral nucleic acid:
   Interferons bind to surface receptors and induce the synthesis of inhibitory proteins which interfere with translation of viral mRNA to viral protein.

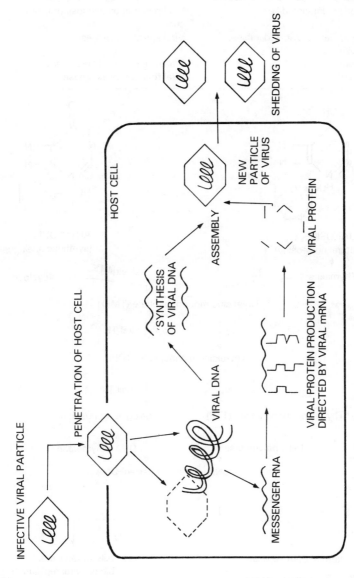

Fig. 20.10 The virus replication cycle.

Table 20.6 Antiviral drugs

Examples	Actions
Amantadine; Rimantadine	Viral penetration and loss of protein coat
Acyclovir; Ganciclovir; Vidarabine; Idoxuridine	Viral specific enzymes
Interferons	Translation of viral nucleic acid
Zidovudine	Viral reverse transcriptase

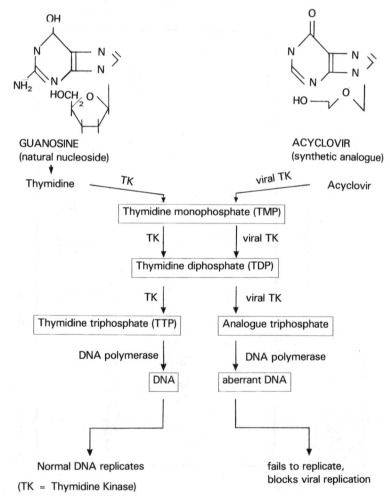

GUANOSINE
(natural nucleoside)

ACYCLOVIR
(synthetic analogue)

Thymidine — *TK* → viral TK — Acyclovir

Thymidine monophosphate (TMP)

TK | viral TK

Thymidine diphosphate (TDP)

TK | viral TK

Thymidine triphosphate (TTP) | Analogue triphosphate

DNA polymerase | DNA polymerase

DNA | aberrant DNA

Normal DNA replicates

fails to replicate, blocks viral replication

(TK = Thymidine Kinase)

Fig. 20.11 Action of acyclovir on nucleic acid synthesis by virally infected cells.

ANTIFUNGALS

Modes of action of antifungals

Polyenes
These bind to membrane ergosterol (fungal) rather than cholesterol (animal) and form a hydrophilic pore. Out of this hole leaks sugar and potassium; acid leaks in and stops enzyme activity. Liposomal amphotericin provides better delivery to the CNS.

Imidazoles
These inhibit ergosterol synthesis. This leads to a leaking membrane of fungal cell, which allows a lethal accumulation of peroxide.
   Miconazole also inhibits ATPase in yeasts. Ketoconazole may reduce the synthesis of testosterone and glucocorticoids in man.

Triazoles
Selective inhibitor of fungal enzymes necessary for the synthesis of ergosterol.

Miscellaneous
Flucytosine enters the fungal cell under the stimulus of cytosine permease. It is then converted by deaminase to 5-fluorouracil which is incorporated into fungal RNA and hence inhibits its function.
   Griseofulvin inhibits assembly of fungal microtubules and causes stunting and branching of hyphae.
   Benzoic acid is uncharged in the extracellular fluid and can in this form enter the fungal cell. The benzoate ion within the cytoplasm inhibits fungal phosphofructokinase.

Table 20.7 Antifungal drugs

Type	Examples	Uses
POLYENES	Amphotericin	Candida; aspergillus; mucor; blastomyces
	Nystatin	Candida; histoplasma; cryptococcus
	Natamycin	Candida
IMIDAZOLES	Clotrimazole	Candida; dermatophytes
	Econazole	Candida; dermatophytes
	Miconazole	Candida; dermatophytes
	Ketoconazole	Candida; dermatophytes
TRIAZOLES	Fluconazole	Candida; cryptococcus
	Itraconazole	Candida; dermatophytes
MISCELLANEOUS	5-fluorocytosine	Candida; cryptococcus
	Griseofulvin	Dermatophytes
	Benzoic acid	Dermatophytes
	Undecenoates	Dermatopyhtes
	Tolnaftate	Dermatophytes

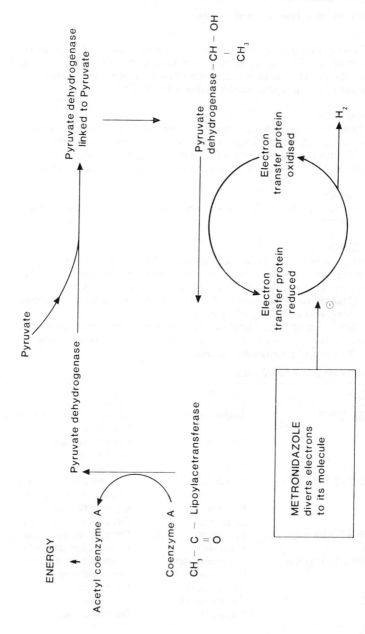

Fig. 20.12 Mode of action of metronidazole.

Table 20.8 Drugs used in the treatment of intestinal parasitic diseases

Drug	Action	Pharmacokinetics	Toxicity	Principal uses
METRONIDAZOLE	Inhibition of anaerobic electron transfer energy production.	Well absorbed from gut. Excreted in bile, urine and saliva.	Frequently produces metallic taste. Nausea. Antabuse reaction. Unusually produces dizziness, numbness, headache and neuropathy.	Tissue invasive and dysenteric amoebiasis. Giardia lamblia. (Also used in Trichomonas vaginalis and anaerobic infections).
PIPERAZINE	Blocks acetylcholine in motor end plate of worms and produces flaccid paralysis. Also stimulates inhibitory receptors.	Well absorbed from gut— but still affects gut parasites.	Toxicity uncommon: nausea, diarrhoea, aggravation of epilepsy. High levels give neuromuscular blockade, confusion and incoordination.	Ascaris lumbricoides. Enterobius vermicularis.
PYRANTEL PAMOATE	Affects neuromuscular junction in worms and gives a spastic paralysis.	Little absorbed from gut.	Well tolerated—but 50% patients experience some dizziness, drowsiness and GI disturbances.	Ascaris lumbricoides; Hookworms; Enterobius vermicularis.
THIABENDAZOLE	Kills developing worms by enzyme inhibition Specifically inhibits helminth fumarase.	Well absorbed from gut and enters tissues (thus effective in cutaneous larva migrans). Rapidly excreted in urine.	Side effects common: dizziness and GI disturbances.	Broad spectrum anthelmintic, and drug of choice in strongyloidiasis.
PYRVINIUM PAMOATE	Depletes carbohydrate energy stores in worm.	Little absorbed from gut.	Well tolerated, but some dizziness and GI disturbances.	Enterobius vermicularis.

(contd)

Table 20.8 (contd)

Drug	Action	Pharmacokinetics	Toxicity	Principal uses
NICLOSAMIDE	Inhibition of oxidative phosphorylation in worm mitochondria. Scolex released and worm digested.	Not absorbed from gut.	Well tolerated.	Drug of choice for tapeworms.
MEBENDAZOLE	Inhibition of glucose uptake by helminths with consequent depletion of ATP.	Little absorbed from gut.	Well tolerated.	Broadest spectrum of antihelmintic activity: *Trichiuris trichiuria*; Hookworms; *Ascaris lumbricoides*; *Enterobius vermicularis*; Cestodes (in large doses).
LEVAMISOLE	Paralyses worms by ganglion stimulation. Also inhibits helminth fumarate reductase (in the host T lymphocytes are stimulated).	Well absorbed from gut.	Low toxicity in recommended doses.	*Ascaris lumbricoides*, Hookworms, (also under trial for treatment of immunodeficiency states and neoplasms).
BEPHENIUM	Stimulates cholinergic receptor of the worm followed by irreversible paralysis.	Little absorbed from gut.	Frequent toxicity: GI disturbances, headache, dizziness, hypotension.	Hookworms; *Ascaris lumbricoides*.
DILOXANIDE	Kills *E. histolytica* trophozoites, on direct contact.	Little absorbed from gut.	No toxicity reported.	Used in asymptomatic amoebiasis.
PRAZIQUANTEL	Stimulates movement of worm and paralyses suckers. Worm loses grip. Increased susceptibility to proteolytic enzymes	Well absorbed from gut. Rapid metabolism.	Well tolerated.	Drug of choice in schistosomiasis.

IMMUNOGLOBULINS

Intravenous administration of antibody may offer short-term protection (few weeks) against an infection or toxic product. The antibody used may be polyclonal anti-serum from normal or hyperimmune human serum or a monoclonal antibody.

Infection or toxin	Source of antibody	Uses
Hepatitis A	Pooled human serum	Protection against infection during travel
Rubella	Normal human serum	Protection after exposure to rubella
Hepatitis B	Hyperimmune human serum	Protection after exposure to virus
Rabies	Hyperimmune human serum	Following a bite by a rabid animal
Varicella zoster	Hyperimmune human serum	After exposure in an immunocompromised patient
Cytomegalovirus (CMV)	Hyperimmune human serum	Life-or-sight threatening CMV infection in an immunocompromised patient
Bacterial lipopolysaccharide (endotoxin)	Monoclonal antibody against endotoxin	Gram-negative septicaemia (role not yet established)
Tumour necrosis factor; produced by host in response to infection	Monoclonal antibody	Septicaemic shock (role not yet established)

21. Anticancer drugs

Classification
1. Alkylating agents
2. Antimetabolites
3. Plant alkaloids
4. Anti-tumour antibiotics
5. Other antineoplastic drugs
6. Hormones
7. Biological response modifiers.

Many of these drugs interfere with cell replication by blocking nucleotide synthesis and so act preferentially on dividing cells. Thus not only are malignant tumours affected, but the following proliferating tissues may be damaged:

1. Bone marrow (red cell, leucocyte and platelet formation)
2. Gonads (production of germ cells; infertility; premature menopause)
3. Gastrointestinal tract (maintenance of the epithelial lining)
4 Skin (particularly the bases of the hair follicles: produces reversible alopecia).

THE CELL CYCLE

Cells may exist in a number of distinct phases.

Anticancer drugs usually inhibit or destroy cells in the proliferative phases. Some (e.g. alkylating agents) are cycle specific and act on cells at all stages of proliferation, whilst others (e.g. methotrexate, 6–mercaptopurine and vinca alkaloids) are phase specific and act mainly at a certain phase of the cell cycle. A few show no specificity for cells in cycle and are equally toxic to resting (G_0) and dividing cells.

For each drug, the percentage kill of tumour cell is associated with killing of normal cells, i.e. therapeutic indices differ. Non–cycle dependent drugs have little differential toxicity for tumour cells so they are highly toxic and total dose determines effect. Phase specific agents act only on cells actually in the sensitive phase of the cycle so killing reaches a plateau and cell kill is not increased by using larger doses. Cycle specific agents may kill more tumour cells if dose is increased although toxicity may be unacceptable at high doses.

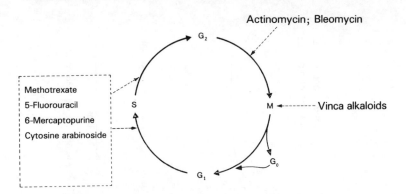

G₀ — quiescent, non-dividing (resting) phase
G₁ — prereplicative phase
S   — DNA replication   ⎤
G₂ — postreplicative phase. Preparation for cell division   ⎬ proliferative phases
M   — mitosis (prophase, metaphase, anaphase, telophase)   ⎦

Fig. 21.1

Slow growing tumours (with many cells in G_0 phase) are unlikely to be
eradicated by phase or cycle dependent drugs.

Many tumour cells grow rapidly but this is not a uniform
characteristic. Their growth rates vary and overlap normal tissues.

Small tumours often contain more rapidly dividing cells than large
ones and may then be susceptible to chemotherapy. Therefore, on
occasions tumours are surgically debulked before drugs are given.

SOME PRINCIPLES OF CANCER CHEMOTHERAPY

1. Cure probably requires complete eradication of tumour cells
2. A given dose of drug kills a given percentage of malignant cells in
   unit time. Thus number of cells before therapy determines the
   number of cells surviving therapy. The earlier treatment is started
   and the smaller the tumour, the better the result
3. Clinical manifestations of cancer occur at a time of considerable
   tumour burden. Thus treatment may need to be prolonged if cure
   is intended
4. Treatment is a balance between the toxic effects of the drugs
   (particularly on the bone marrow) and their efficacy
5. Curative chemotherapy must reduce tumour cells to nil or to such
   low numbers that body defences can kill the rest. Aim is to allow
   more rapid recovery of normal cells whilst killing cancer cells by
   pulsed therapy

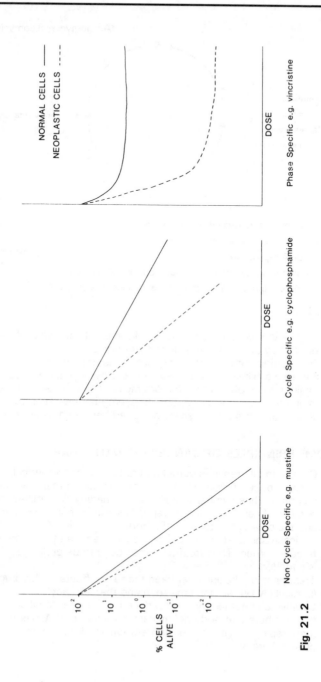

Fig. 21.2

6. Adjuvant therapy (cytotoxic drugs given after primary treatment of cancer by surgery or radiotherapy) to eradicate seedling metastases is undergoing clinical evaluation. Of value in some patients with breast cancer.

Cytotoxic chemotherapy is potentially curative in leukaemia, lymphoma, testicular tumours, choriocarcinoma and embryonal childhood tumours. Other chemoresponsive but not usually chemocurable tumours include small cell lung cancer, ovarian cancer and myeloma. Chemotherapy has a palliative role in breast cancer.

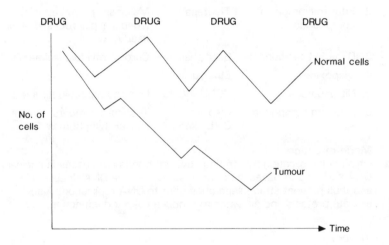

Fig. 21.3

ALKYLATING AGENTS

Group	Drug	Uses (examples)
1. Mustards	Mustine	Lymphomas
	Chlorambucil	Chronic lymphatic leukaemia and lymphomas
	Melphalan	Myelomatosis
	Cyclophosphamide	Lymphomas
	Ifosfamide	Leukaemias
	(activated by liver to alkylating metabolites)	Carcinoma of breast, Sarcoma

Cyclophosphamide and ifosfamide are metabolised to acrolein which is toxic to bladder and kidneys and limits the dose which can be given unless mesna (mercaptoethane sulphonate sodium) is simultaneously administered. This enters only the renal tubules (and so does not affect cytotoxic effects) where it forms a stable non-irritant thio–ether with acrolein.

$$CH_2CHCHO + HSCH_2CH_2SO_3Na \rightarrow NaSO_3CH_2CH_2SCHCHCHO$$
Acrolein   Mesna   Stable thio–ether

Mustards also used in combination chemotherapy for a number of solid tumours.

2. Ethyleneimmonium compounds	Thiotepa	Malignant pleural effusion (chemical pleurodesis)—little used now
3. Dimethyl sulphonates	Busulphan	Chronic myeloid leukaemia
4. Diepoxides	Ethoglucid	
5. Nitrosoureas	CCNU, BCNU	Lymphoma; brain tumours
6. Platinum compounds	Cisplatin Carboplatin	Testicular tumours; ovarian cancer; lymphomas

Mode of action
Inhibit cell replication by forming covalent bonds with bases in nuclear DNA and bind to bases in opposite strands of the DNA double helix and thus prevent strand separation prior to DNA replication. Also alkylate proteins and enzymes to produce cellular dysfunction.

Toxicity
Cisplatin—nephrotoxic and ototoxic and causes severe nausea and vomiting

Carboplatin—well tolerated; myelosuppressive

ANTIMETABOLITES

Group	Drug	Uses
1. Folic acid antagonists	Methotrexate	Acute lymphoblastic leukaemia Lymphomas Chorioncarcinoma Solid tumours, e.g. osteogenic sarcoma
2. Purine antagonists	6-mercaptopurine 6-thioguanine	Acute leukaemias Acute leukaemias

3. Pyrimidine antagonists	5-fluorodeoxyuridine 5-fluorouracil }	Adenocarcinomas of the gastrointestinal tract Carcinoma of breast and ovary
	6-azauracil 6-azauridine }	Acute leukaemias
	Cytosine arabinoside	Acute myeloblastic leukaemia

Modes of action

Methotrexate analogue of folic acid	Irreversible inhibition of dihydrofolate reductase which blocks the reaction uridylate → thymidylate due to the failure of formation of active folate to act as a methyl group carrier.
6-mercaptopurine (6MP) analogue of adenine	6MP is converted to the 5'-phosphate nucleotide (thioinosinate) which blocks purine synthesis at several steps (including; IMP → adenylosuccinate; synthesis of guanylate; glutamine + PRPP → ribosylamine-5'-phosphate).
5-fluorouracil (5FU) analogue of uracil	5FU is converted to the 5'-phosphate nucleotide (F-UMP) and then to the deoxynucleotide (5-dUMP). The latter inhibits thymidylate synthetase.
Cytosine arabinoside (Cytarabine) analogue of cytidine	Cytarabine is converted to the 5'-phosphate nucleotide (ara-CTP) which inhibits nucleoside diphosphate reductase and RNA-dependent DNA polymerase (reverse transcriptase).
6-thioguanine analogue of guanine	Incorporated into DNA in place of guanine.

PLANT ALKALOIDS

Vinca alkaloids (from periwinkle): vincristine; vinblastine; vindesine

Mode of action
Bind to microtubules and disrupt spindle formation so chromosomes do not separate at mitosis. Affect other microtubular functions (e.g. membrane mobility and transport) and enzyme activity.

Vincristine —toxicity: mainly peripheral neuropathy
          —uses: leukaemia, lymphomas, neuroblastoma, sarcoma
Vinblastine—toxicity: mainly myelosuppression
          —uses: lymphomas, breast cancer, chorionepithelioma

Etoposide (from May Apple)

Mode of action
Spindle poison but not by binding to microtubules; blocks DNA
synthesis.

Uses
Lymphomas, small cell lung cancer, leukaemia.

ANTITUMOUR ANTIBIOTICS

Anthracyclines
Doxorubicin (Adriamycin); daunorubicin; epirubicin.

Mode of action
Intercalate DNA helix thus uncoiling and preventing DNA and RNA
synthesis. Also damage cell membrane and form free radicles which
peroxidise lipids.
   Main problems: locally irritant (if given outside vein by accident);
alopecia; dose-related cardiotoxicity.

Uses
Lymphoma, breast cancer, leukaemia.

Actinomycin

Mode of action .
DNA intercalation to inhibit RNA synthesis.

Uses
Wilm's tumour of kindey (children), chorioncarcinoma, embryonal
rhabdomyo-sarcoma.

Bleomycin (mixture of polypeptides)

Mode of action
Fragments DNA and inhibits thymidine incorporation into DNA.
   Main problems: pulmonary fibrosis, acute flu-like illness after
injection; pigmentation of skin.

Uses
Lymphomas, testicular teratomas, cancer of head and neck.

OTHER ANTI–NEOPLASTIC DRUGS

Mitozantrone
An anthracenedione resembling an anthracycline which acts as an
intercalating agent but has less cardiotoxicity, causes less alopecia, is
less irritant but is more myelosuppressive. Used in breast cancer.

Procarbazine
A weak MAO inhibitor.
Mode of action
Depolymerizes DNA—probable alkylating agent.
Uses
Hodgkin's lymphoma.

Etoposide
Epipodophyllotoxin (synthetic derivative of podophyllotoxin).
Mode of action
Causes single strand DNA breaks and inhibits replication.
Toxicity
Myelosuppression dose limiting; alopecia.

L–asparaginase
An enzyme produced by *E. coli.*
Mode of action
Some tumour (unlike normal) cells cannot synthesise asparagine.
Colaspase hydrolyses free tissue and plasma asparagine so depriving
tumours of exogenous amino acid.
Uses
Acute leukaemia.

HORMONES

May produce remission in some cancers but do not eradicate disease.
1. Oestrogen used for two cancers which are partially hormone–
   dependent
   a. Prostatic carcinoma—oestrogens e.g. diethylstiboestrol block
      androgen production with remission in 60% patients with
      advanced disease
   b. Breast cancer—oestrogens give remission in 30% women with
      advanced disease who are 5 years post–menopausal but may
      exacerbate disease in younger women. Tumours with
      oestrogen receptors 6 times more likely to respond (60%) than
      receptor negative tumours (10%)

2. Anti-oestrogens for breast cancer
   a. Tamoxifen—competes with oestradiol for cytoplasmic receptor.
      Few side effects
   b. Aminoglutethimide produces medical adrenalectomy by
      inhibiting adrenal steroid synthesis and inhibits peripheral tissue
      aromatisation of androgens to oestrogens

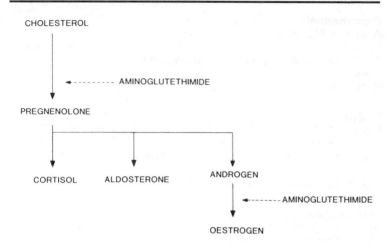

Fig. 21.4

Given with cortisone acetate (replaces cortisol) and fludrocortisone alternate days (replaces aldosterone deficit). Produces sedation, ataxia, dizziness (dose dependent and reduces with chronic therapy—self–induction of metabolising enzymes). Used for breast and prostatic cancer

3. Progestogens, e.g. medroxyprogesterone acetate (Depo–Provera). May produce remission in up to 30% breast cancer resistant to other hormones. Also used in endometrial carcinoma. No side–effects
4. Anti–androgens
   Cyproterone acetate, flutamide for prostatic cancer
5. LHRH analogues
   Leuprorelin, goserelin, buserelin. Equivalent in effectiveness to oestrogens in prostatic carcinoma, with less toxicity
6. Glucocorticoids
   Inhibit lymphoid proliferation. Adverse effects numerous. Used in acute and chronic lymphocytic leukaemia; multiple myeloma; Hodgkin's and non-Hodgkin's lymphomas; breast carcinoma.

BIOLOGICAL RESPONSE MODIFIERS

1. Immunotherapy
   Specific antitumour monoclonal and polyclonal antibody targeting. Under intensive investigation for many tumour types
2. Lymphokines
   Interferon—natural antiviral substances. Effective in hairy cell leukaemia; also being investigated in renal carcinoma, CML and myeloma

3. IL2 (± Lymphokine-activated killer (LAK) cells)
   Modulation of the immune response under investigation in renal
   carcinoma. Toxicity due to vascular leak and multiple organ failure
4. Growth factors
   Haemopoietic growth factors (G-CSF, CM-CSF, IL3) are being
   tested to reduce myelosuppression with cytotoxic drugs
5. Other
   Intensive search for specific growth factor receptor agonists and
   antagonists and antisense oligonucleotides to modulate individual
   tumour proliferation.

Toxic effects of cancer chemotherapy
Major problems due to inability of drug action to differentiate normal
from neoplastic cells.
1. Bone marrow: leucopenia; thrombocytopenia; rarely anaemia or
   total aplasia. Causes infection and bleeding
2. GI tract: ulceration of mouth and intestine, diarrhoea
3. Testis: azoospermia and infertility
4. Ovary: infertility; premature menopause
5. Hair follicles: alopecia
6. Local irritation: some drugs cause ulceration if extravasated during
   injection
7. Vomiting: major problem with some drugs, e.g. cisplatin, CCNU,
   doxorubicin.

Longer term hazards of cancer chemotherapy
1. Gonadal damage—alkylating agents, vinca, alkaloids, cytosine
   arabinoside. Azoospermia usual during treatment. Recovery often
   occurs but may take several years (N.B. many patients have low
   sperm count before treatment). Many women develop
   amenorrhoea after cytotoxic drugs but periods restart when
   treatment stopped. Women may have premature menopause.
2. Second malignancy e.g. after treatment of Hodgkins lymphoma
   with radio- and chemotherapy incidence of acute leukaemia
   increased.
3. Teratogenesis: avoid pregnancy for at least 4 months after end of
   treatment.

ACQUIRED TUMOUR RESISTANCE TO CYTOTOXIC AGENTS

Mechanism	Examples.
1. Reduced uptake of drug	Methotrexate; Daunorubicin
2. Deletion of enzyme to activate drug	Cytosine arabinoside; 5-fluorouracil
3. Increased detoxication of drug	6-mercaptopurine
4. Increased concentration of target enzyme	Methotrexate
5. Decreased requirement for specific metabolic product	Asparaginase
6. Increased utilisation of alternative metabolic pathways	Antimetabolites
7. Rapid repair of drug-induced lesion	Alkylating agents
8. Decreased number of receptors for drug	Hormones
9. Alteration in proliferation rate. ?underlying mechanism.	Myeloma, chronic myeloid leukaemia commonly terminate in a more aggressive phase.

Index

NB Page numbers in *italics* refer to figures and tables.

246   Index